TRUE JU

Papa, I'm Hungry

50 Simple Meals Your Child Can Prepare Daily

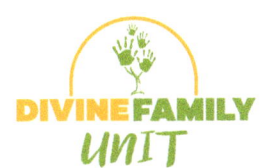

First published by Divine Family Unit, LLC 2023

Copyright © 2023 by True Ju

All rights reserved. No part of this publication may be reproduced, stored or transmitted in any form or by any means, electronic, mechanical, photocopying, recording, scanning, or otherwise without written permission from the publisher. It is illegal to copy this book, post it to a website, or distribute it by any other means without permission.

True Ju asserts the moral right to be identified as the author of this work.

True Ju has no responsibility for the persistence or accuracy of URLs for external or third-party Internet Websites referred to in this publication and does not guarantee that any content on such Websites is, or will remain, accurate or appropriate.

Designations used by companies to distinguish their products are often claimed as trademarks. All brand names and product names used in this book and on its cover are trade names, service marks, trademarks and registered trademarks of their respective owners. The publishers and the book are not associated with any product or vendor mentioned in this book. None of the companies referenced within the book have endorsed the book.

Disclaimer -

"Papa, I'm Hungry: 50 Simple Meals Your Child Can Prepare Daily" is an innovative children's cookbook that empowers young chefs aged 10-16 to explore the joy of cooking and create nutritious meals. While we have taken every effort to ensure the safety and age-appropriateness of the recipes provided, it is essential to emphasize that adult supervision is still required during the cooking process.

Parents and guardians must exercise caution and oversee their children while the young chefs prepare the recipes in this cookbook. Cooking involves the use of sharp utensils, hot surfaces, and potentially hazardous kitchen tools, and accidents may occur despite the utmost care.

The authors, publishers, and vendors of "Papa, I'm Hungry" hold no responsibility for any accidents, injuries, damages, or losses that may arise from implementing the recipes or using the techniques outlined in the book. The responsibility for ensuring a safe and supervised cooking environment lies solely with the parents or guardians.

We urge parents to teach their young chefs about kitchen safety, appropriate handling of kitchen tools, and the potential risks associated with cooking. Through mindful guidance and supervision, parents can ensure a positive and rewarding cooking experience for their children while fostering their culinary skills and confidence.

Parents acknowledge and accept their responsibility for monitoring and supervising their child's cooking activities using this cookbook. As such, "Papa, I'm Hungry" becomes a delightful resource to nurture a love for cooking, while ensuring safety remains a top priority in the kitchen.

Images Disclaimer -

All images were staged and captured by True Ju for the exclusive use of Divine Family Unit, LLC, ©2023 - All Rights Reserved.

First edition

ISBN: 979-8-98-657365-6

Advisor: Divine Family Unit, LLC

This book was professionally typeset on Reedsy.
Find out more at reedsy.com

This cookbook is dedicated to those who want to grow up and take their youthfulness along for the ride.

Contents

Foreword		iii
Preface		v
1	Veggie Omelet with Whole-Grain Toast	1
2	Greek Yogurt Parfait with Fresh Fruits and Granola	7
3	Grilled Cheese Sandwich with Tomato Soup	11
4	Veggie Wraps with Hummus	17
5	Chicken and Vegetable Stir-Fry	23
6	Peanut Butter and Banana Sandwich on Whole-Grain Bread	28
7	Fruit Salad with a Drizzle of Honey	32
8	Turkey and Cheese Roll-Ups	36
9	Avocado Toast with a Sprinkle of Sesame Seeds	40
10	Tuna Salad Lettuce Wraps	44
11	Quinoa Salad with Veggies and Feta Cheese	49
12	Veggie Sushi Rolls	53
13	Baked Sweet Potato Fries	58
14	Spinach and Feta Stuffed Chicken Breast	63
15	Baked Salmon with Lemon and Herbs	68
16	Whole-Grain Pasta with Marinara Sauce and Veggies	73
17	Fruit Smoothie with Yogurt and Spinach	78
18	Stuffed Bell Peppers with Lean Ground Turkey	83
19	Veggie and Cheese Quesadillas	87
20	Mediterranean Chickpea Salad	91
21	Turkey and Vegetable Kebabs	95
22	Broccoli and Cheese Stuffed Potatoes	99
23	Hummus and Veggie Platter	103
24	Mini Turkey Meatloaf with Mashed Cauliflower	106

25	Brown Rice with Black Beans and Salsa	111
26	Zucchini Noodles with Tomato Sauce	115
27	Grilled Chicken Caesar Salad	119
28	Fruit Kabobs with Yogurt Dip	123
29	Lentil Soup with Vegetables	127
30	Baked Tilapia with a Side of Steamed Broccoli	132
31	Veggie-Loaded Pizza on Whole-Grain Crust	136
32	Stuffed Mushrooms with Spinach and Cheese	140
33	Fruit and Yogurt Popsicles	144
34	Teriyaki Tofu with Rice and Steamed Veggies	148
35	Egg Salad Lettuce Cups	152
36	Cucumber and Cream Cheese Sandwiches	156
37	Quinoa-Stuffed Bell Peppers	160
38	Veggie and Cheese Frittata	165
39	Baked Chicken Tenders with Sweet Potato Wedges	170
40	Caprese Salad with Balsamic Glaze	174
41	Veggie Chili with Cornbread	178
42	Baked Falafel with Tahini Dressing	184
43	Greek Salad with Olives and Feta Cheese	189
44	Cauliflower Crust Pizza with Veggie Toppings	193
45	Chicken and Vegetable Kebabs	198
46	Veggie-Loaded Macaroni and Cheese	202
47	Banana and Almond Butter Smoothie	206
48	Veggie and Cheese Stuffed Mushrooms	210
49	Black Bean and Corn Salad	215
50	Turkey and Avocado Lettuce Wraps	219
51	Conclusion	224
About the Author		227

Foreword

Welcome to **"Papa, I'm Hungry: 50 Simple Meals Your Child Can Prepare Daily"** – a cookbook born from the hustle and heart of a work-from-home dad determined to nourish his family with quick, tasty meals amidst the whirlwind of responsibilities. Within these pages lies a tale of dedication, family bonds, and the joy of watching young chefs blossom in the kitchen.

In the early days of my marriage, as the day's responsibilities piled up, I found myself multitasking from dawn to dusk. Balancing work, sales calls, property management, and everything in between, while my wife juggled her demanding career in the banking industry. Amidst this hustle, a familiar phrase echoed through our home: "Papa…I'm hungry."

As a work-driven individual, time slipped away unnoticed, making the need for quick and healthy meals a must. The idea of my boys cooking for themselves someday briefly crossed my mind, but in the rush of life, it remained fleeting. Living in the moment, I was determined to face each challenge head-on.

Through trial and error, I crafted a system that allowed me to prepare simple, fun, and speedy meals that the boys loved, and their energy levels appreciated. No after-school programs or daycare—our family embraced activities together, like martial arts and basketball, cherishing every moment we shared.

Success arrived when I discovered that simplicity was the key. These early culinary endeavors left a lasting impact; my sons, now teenagers, confidently experiment in the kitchen, drawing from their experiences of tasting and preparing delicious meals. They offer their culinary creations to their siblings, their mother, and me, just as I once did for them.

And so, we are thrilled to share this journey with you and your family. Inside these pages, you'll find a treasure trove of recipes, meticulously crafted with young chefs in mind. Empower your children to embrace the joy of cooking, cultivating skills that will enrich their lives both at home and beyond.

Let these recipes be the bridge that connects your family, where food preparation becomes a delightful experience, and the dining table becomes a gathering place of love and laughter. As a Divine Family Unit, you'll witness your children bloom into confident and skilled young chefs, ready to take on life's adventures.

So, dive in and savor the delicious rewards that await you. From our family to yours, may these recipes nourish your hearts and souls, and may the culinary journey be filled with moments to cherish forever. Enjoy!

Preface

Welcome to "**Papa, I'm Hungry: 50 Simple Meals Your Child Can Prepare Daily**," an innovative cookbook designed to empower young chefs aged 10-16 and provide busy parents with a solution for healthy meals amidst their work constraints. Within these pages, you'll find clear and age-appropriate recipe instructions, complemented by motivating quotes, all crafted to help your aspiring young chefs feel confident in the kitchen.

At Divine Family Unit, we understand the challenges faced by parents striving to provide nutritious meals for their children while juggling busy schedules. With our firsthand experience as parents, Coach Rae and Coach True Ju, a loving couple of 15 years, and parents to four beautiful children, realized the importance of creating a cookbook that not only supports healthful eating but also empowers young chefs to take charge in the kitchen.

We know how daunting it can be to keep schedules and complete daily tasks while ensuring your family receives the healthiest meals possible. "Papa, I'm Hungry" presents a curated collection of delicious and wholesome recipes that we have seamlessly integrated into our daily routines. These are the very recipes that have nourished and delighted our own family.

Each recipe in this cookbook is not only chosen for its nutritional value but also for its simplicity and ease of preparation. We believe that cooking should be a joyful experience, fostering a sense of creativity and accomplishment in your children as they embark on their culinary journey.

As you dive into the pages of "Papa, I'm Hungry," you'll discover a treasury of delightful recipes and uplifting motivational quotes, inspiring your young chefs to embrace the joy of cooking. We hope this book serves as a valuable tool in your household, allowing your children to step confidently into the kitchen while you remain assured of their safety and skill development.

With heartfelt prayers, we present this cookbook to you, trusting that it will assist your family in savoring not only delicious meals but also treasured moments shared around the dining table. May your culinary adventure be filled with love, laughter, and the joy of creating lifelong memories together. Bon appétit!

1

Veggie Omelet with Whole-Grain Toast

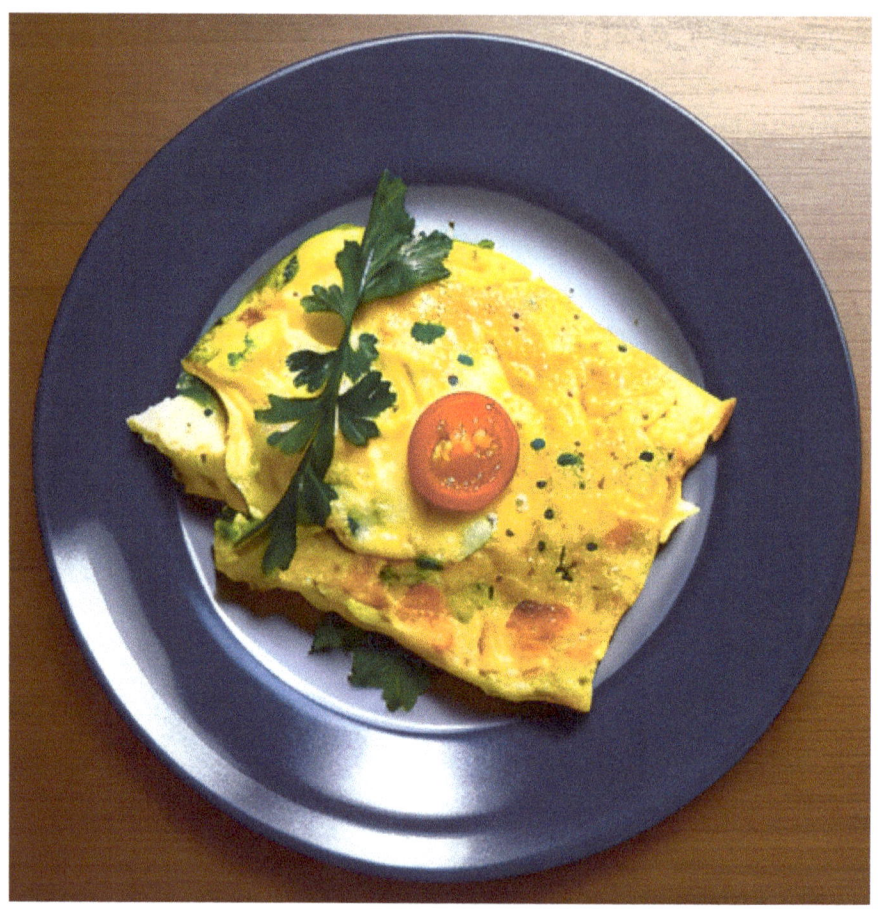

Veggie Omelet

VEGGIE OMELET WITH WHOLE-GRAIN TOAST

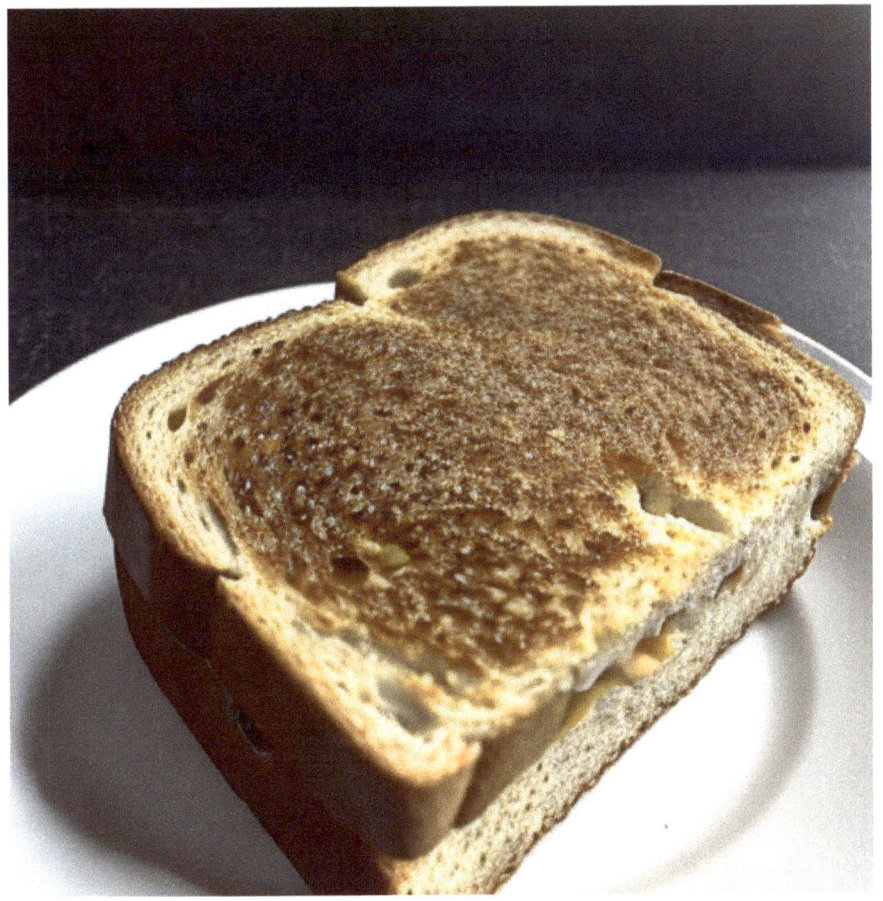

Whole Grain Toast

"*Every great chef started with a simple recipe and a curious heart. Embrace the kitchen adventure, and soon you'll create masterpieces of your own.*" - *Divine Family Unit*

In the early years of our culinary adventure, my sons were young, and their tastes were still underdeveloped. I knew I needed to create meals that they would genuinely enjoy while ensuring they received the nutrition they needed to thrive. The Veggie Omelet with Whole-Grain Toast became a breakfast favorite that ticked all the right boxes.

One bright morning, as the sun peeked over the horizon, my sons burst into the kitchen, their enthusiasm palpable. They were eager to take charge of the breakfast preparations, and I happily obliged, guiding them every step of the way.

As we cracked the eggs into the mixing bowl, I explained that eggs were a fantastic source of protein, vital for their growing bodies. Watching them whisk the eggs with excitement, I introduced the vibrant colors of diced bell peppers, cherry tomatoes, and baby spinach, chosen for their nutrients and vibrant flavors.

As the omelet sizzled in the pan, filling the kitchen with a mouthwatering aroma, I showed them how the chosen vegetables provided essential vitamins and minerals, ensuring they stay strong and healthy.

To complement the omelet, we toasted whole-grain bread, explaining how it contained fiber, promoting good digestion and keeping them full and energized throughout the morning.

Finally, with eager anticipation, they flipped the omelet onto a plate, the colors of the vegetables creating a delightful mosaic. As they savored their creation, I couldn't help but marvel at how far they had come in the kitchen.

From that day on, the Veggie Omelet with Whole-Grain Toast became a breakfast tradition in our home. It was a meal that not only nourished their bodies but also fed their culinary curiosity. As my sons grew older, they continued to prepare this wholesome breakfast, each time with a sense of pride and accomplishment.

This chapter celebrates the joy of simple breakfasts, the delight of colorful vegetables, and the beginning of a culinary journey that has enriched our lives in countless ways. May you and your young chefs savor the same magic as you prepare this Veggie Omelet with Whole-Grain Toast together, nurturing not only their bodies but their love for cooking as well. Bon appétit!

Veggie Omelet with Whole-Grain Toast:

Ingredients:
   - 2 large eggs
   - 1/4 cup chopped veggies (bell peppers, onions, tomatoes, spinach, mushrooms, etc.)
   - 1 tablespoon milk (optional)
   - Salt and pepper to taste
   - 1 teaspoon butter or cooking spray
   - 2 slices of whole-grain bread

Instructions:

1. Wash and chop your favorite veggies. Ask an adult to help with cutting if needed.

2. Crack the eggs into a bowl. Add a pinch of salt and pepper, and the optional milk for a fluffier omelet. Use a fork or whisk to beat the eggs until well combined.

3. Heat a non-stick frying pan over medium heat. Add the butter or use cooking spray to coat the pan.

4. Pour the beaten eggs into the pan. As the eggs start to set, gently lift the edges with a spatula to let the uncooked egg flow underneath.

5. Once the eggs are mostly set, sprinkle the chopped veggies over one-half of the omelet.

6. Carefully fold the other half of the omelet over the veggies to form a

half-moon shape.

7. Cook for another minute or until the omelet is fully set and slightly golden.

8. Toast the whole-grain bread slices until they are lightly browned.

9. Serve the omelet on a plate with the whole-grain toast on the side.

**Encourage young chefs to appreciate the bounty of fresh ingredients in their cooking and to find joy in the creative process. Happy cooking and layering!

2

Greek Yogurt Parfait with Fresh Fruits and Granola

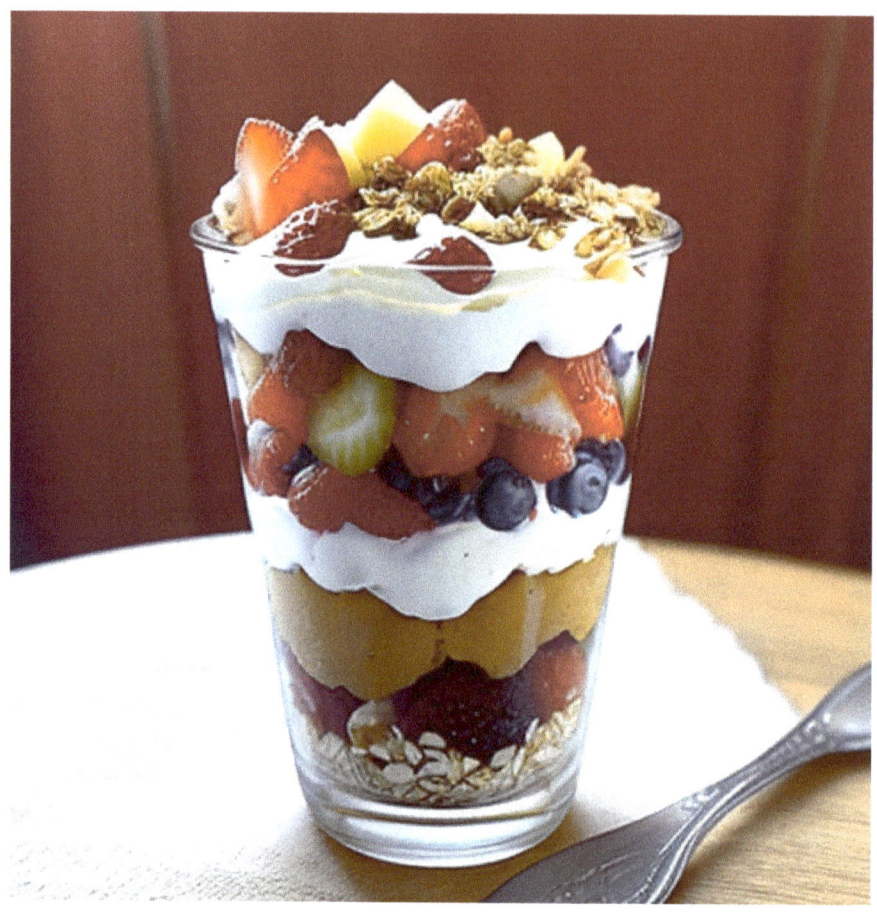

Greek Yogurt Parfait with Fresh Fruits and Granola

"*In cooking and life, every layer adds something special. Embrace the process, and you'll create a masterpiece of flavors and memories.*" - Unknown

In our quest to find delicious and nutritious meals that my sons would love, we stumbled upon a challenge—Greek yogurt. While they adored the crunchy goodness of granola, convincing them to embrace the creamy tang of Greek yogurt was no easy task. But with creativity and a touch of magic, we crafted a delightful solution—the Greek Yogurt Parfait with Fresh Fruits and Granola.

GREEK YOGURT PARFAIT WITH FRESH FRUITS AND GRANOLA

One sunny afternoon, I decided to turn our kitchen into a playful yogurt bar. I laid out an array of colorful bowls filled with fresh, juicy fruits like ripe strawberries, plump blueberries, and succulent peaches, explaining how these fruits were packed with vitamins and antioxidants, perfect for keeping their little bodies strong and healthy.

Next came the star ingredient—Greek yogurt. I introduced them to its creamy texture, subtly emphasizing the protein and probiotics that would support their immune systems and digestion.

But the real fun began when I brought out the beloved granola, crunchy and irresistible. As they sprinkled it atop the yogurt and fruits, their eyes lit up with excitement, realizing that this could be the perfect harmony of flavors they had been searching for.

With a dash of honey drizzled on top, their creation was complete. They eagerly took their first bite, and a symphony of flavors danced on their taste buds. The initial hesitancy toward Greek yogurt was forgotten, replaced by newfound enthusiasm for this delightful parfait.

From that day on, our Greek Yogurt Parfait with Fresh Fruits and Granola became a cherished breakfast and snack option in our home. It was a meal that combined their love for granola with the nourishing goodness of Greek yogurt and a rainbow of fresh fruits.

This chapter celebrates the magic of playful experimentation in the kitchen and the discovery of delightful combinations. As you and your young chefs prepare this Greek Yogurt Parfait with Fresh Fruits and Granola together, may you witness the joy of transformation and the triumph of nutritious choices embraced with open hearts and delighted palates. Bon appétit!

Greek Yogurt Parfait with Fresh Fruits and Granola:

Ingredients:
  - 1 cup Greek yogurt (plain or flavored)
  - Assorted fresh fruits (e.g., berries, sliced bananas, diced mango, etc.)
  - 1/4 cup granola (homemade or store-bought)

Instructions:

1. Wash and prepare the fresh fruits. You can mix and match your favorite fruits or use what's in season.

2. Choose a tall glass or a clear bowl to make the parfait.

3. Start by layering a spoonful of Greek yogurt at the bottom of the glass.

4. Add a layer of your chosen fresh fruits on top of the yogurt.

5. Sprinkle a tablespoon of granola over the fruit layer.

6. Repeat the layers: Greek yogurt, fresh fruits, and granola until you reach the top of the glass.

7. Finish with a final layer of fresh fruits and a small sprinkle of granola for a beautiful presentation.

8. Serve immediately and enjoy your delicious Greek yogurt parfait!

**Encourage young chefs to appreciate the beauty of layering flavors in their cooking and to find joy in the creative process. Happy cooking and layering!

3

Grilled Cheese Sandwich with Tomato Soup

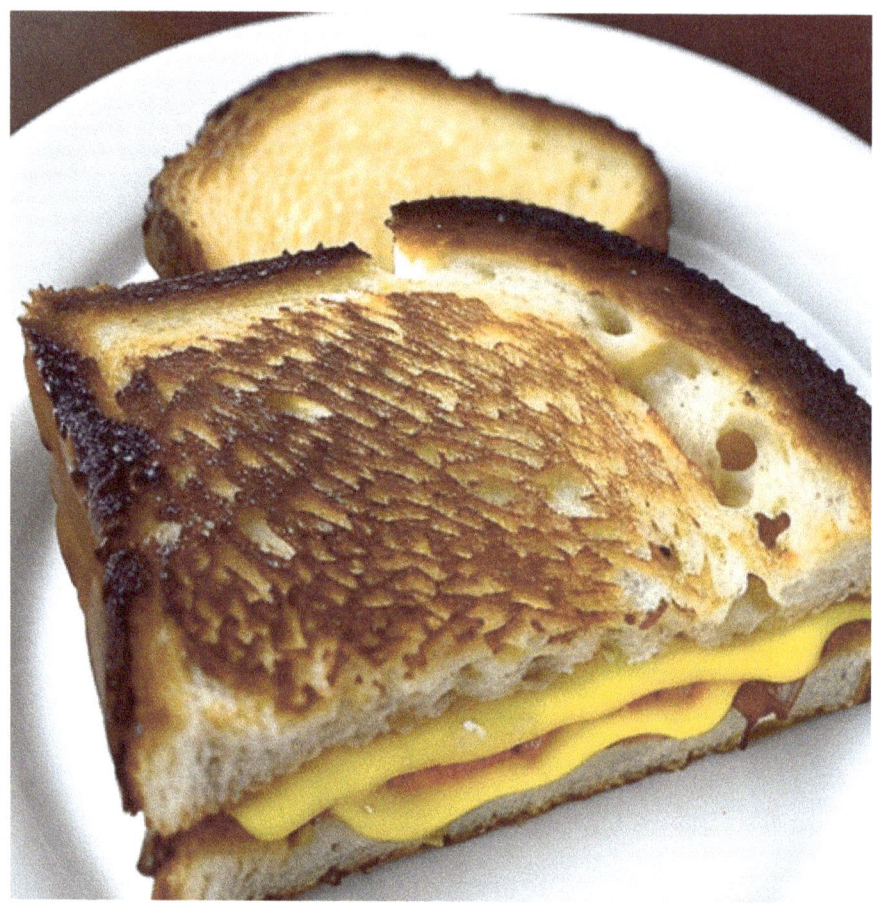
Grilled Cheese Sandwich

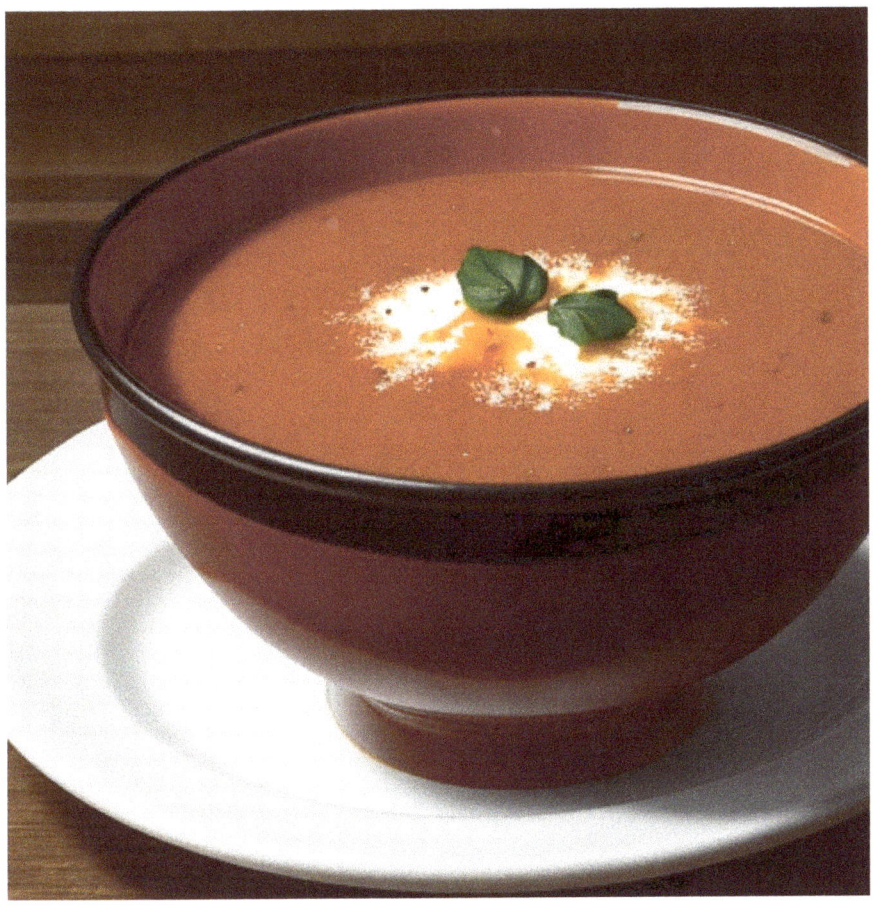

Tomato Soup

"*In every combination, there's a blend of magic. Just like your grilled cheese and tomato soup, embrace the perfect pairing that makes your heart sing!*" - *Papa True Ju*

Ah, the timeless classic that captured my sons' hearts from the very first bite—the Grilled Cheese Sandwich with Tomato Soup. To say they adore this comforting meal would be an understatement; if they had it their way, they'd happily savor it every single day!

It all started on a chilly winter afternoon when we decided to whip up a warm and satisfying lunch together. As we gathered in the kitchen, my sons were already buzzing with excitement, knowing what was on the menu.

We carefully selected the ingredients for our perfect grilled cheese sandwich. Thick slices of crusty bread, lovingly buttered on the outside, and a medley of gooey cheeses that would melt into a velvety embrace with every bite. I explained that the cheese provided essential calcium for their growing bones and teeth, and they giggled at the idea of their sandwiches helping them grow tall and strong.

But no grilled cheese is complete without its perfect companion—tomato soup. We crafted a rich and comforting tomato soup, simmering with ripe tomatoes, aromatic herbs, and a touch of sweetness. I emphasized how the tomatoes were bursting with vitamin C, a powerful nutrient that would help keep them healthy and vibrant.

As we grilled the sandwiches to golden perfection and ladled the steaming soup into bowls, the kitchen was filled with the tantalizing aroma of melted cheese and simmering tomatoes. Their anticipation was palpable, and when the first spoonful of tomato soup met their lips, their faces lit up with delight.

The symphony of flavors between the crispy grilled cheese and the savory tomato soup was pure magic. With each bite, they reveled in the comfort and joy that this simple yet extraordinary meal brought them.

From that moment on, the Grilled Cheese Sandwich with Tomato Soup became an all-time favorite in our household. It was a meal that brought warmth to the coldest days and a smile to their faces like nothing else could.

This chapter celebrates the joy of childhood favorites and the magic of flavors that evoke cherished memories. As you and your young chefs prepare this Grilled Cheese Sandwich with Tomato Soup together, may you revel in the simple pleasures of comfort food and the heartwarming connections it creates around the dining table. Bon appétit!

Grilled Cheese Sandwich with Tomato Soup:

Ingredients:
  - 4 slices of bread (white, whole-grain, or your favorite type)
  - 4 slices of cheese (cheddar, American, or any melting cheese)
  - Butter or margarine (softened)
  - Tomato soup (homemade or store-bought)

Instructions:

1. Lay out the four slices of bread on a clean surface.

2. Place one slice of cheese on two of the bread slices.

3. Close the sandwiches with the other two slices of bread, creating two cheese sandwiches.

4. Spread a thin layer of softened butter or margarine on the outside of each sandwich.

5. Heat a non-stick skillet or griddle over medium heat.

6. Carefully place the sandwiches in the skillet and cook for 2-3 minutes on each side until the bread is golden brown and the cheese is melted.

7. Remove the grilled cheese sandwiches from the skillet and let them cool for a moment.

8. Serve the grilled cheese sandwiches with a side of warm tomato soup for dipping.

**Encourage young chefs to enjoy the comforting harmony of their creations, whether it's in the kitchen or throughout life. Happy cooking and pairing!

4

Veggie Wraps with Hummus

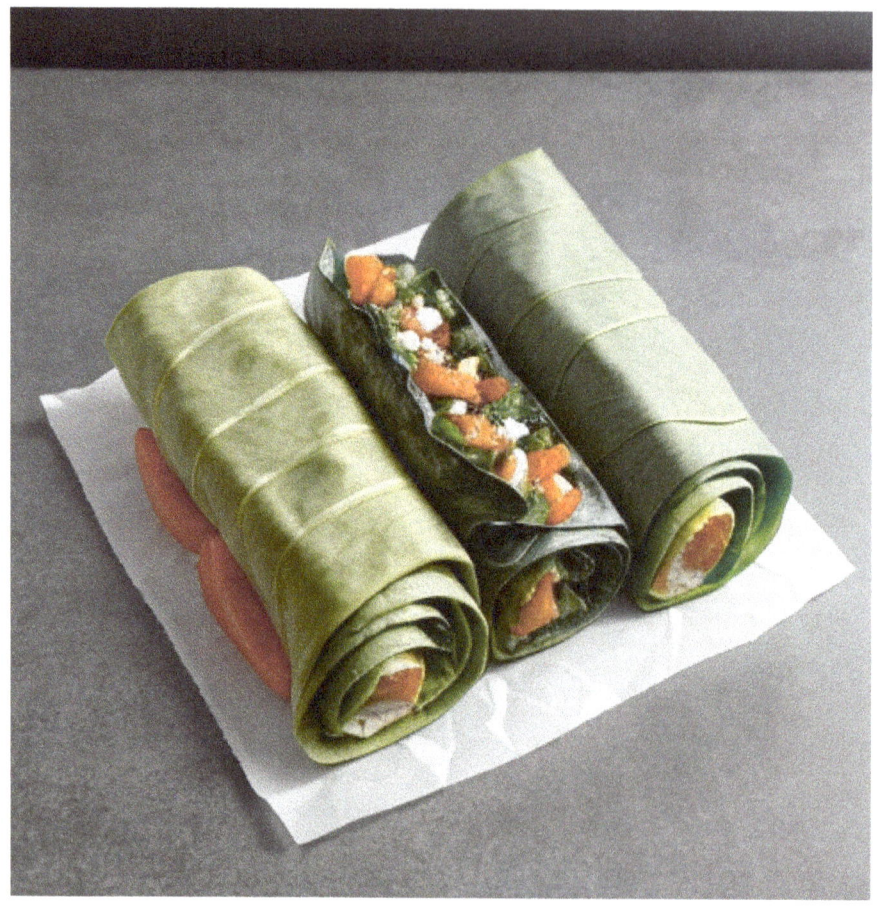

Veggie Wraps

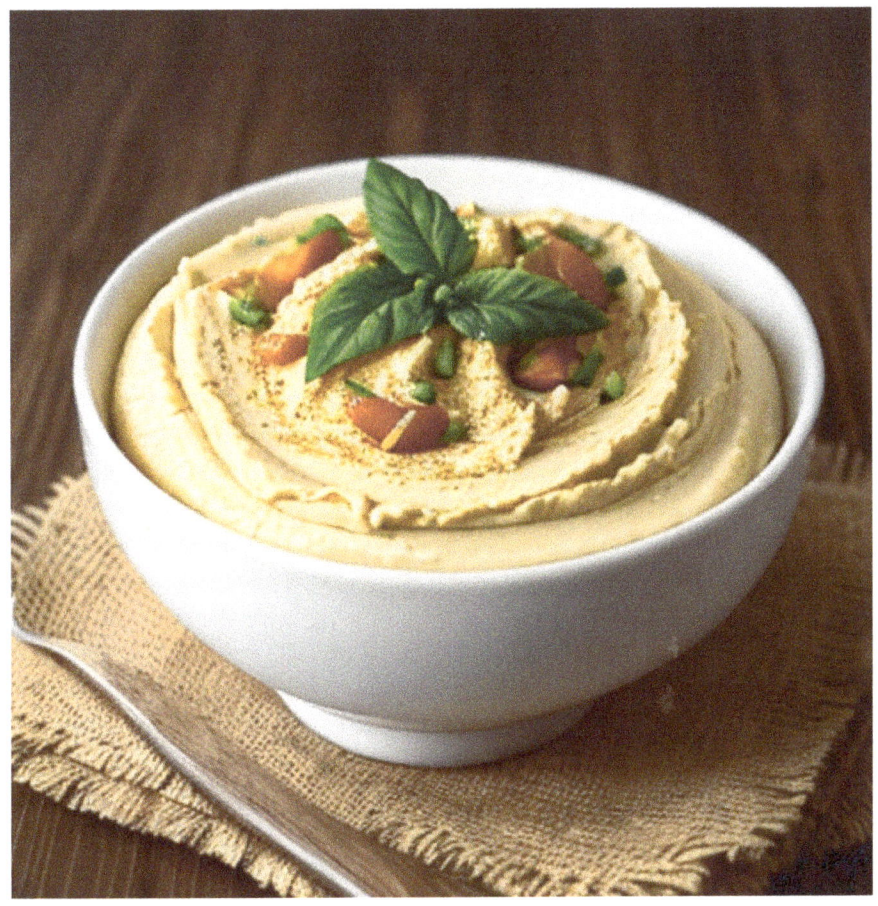

Hummus

"*In every wrap, you hold the power to create a masterpiece of taste and color. Embrace the endless combinations, and let your creativity shine!*" - Coach Rae

In our culinary journey, there was a moment when my sons were met with skepticism about trying new flavors. Enter Veggie Wraps with Hummus—a delightful meal that turned their doubts into wide-eyed wonder, all while celebrating the joy of exploration and discovery.

One sunny afternoon, we embarked on a quest to create a meal that embraced the vibrant colors and flavors of fresh vegetables. As we gathered around the kitchen counter, I introduced them to hummus—an ingredient derived from chickpeas, a food they loved to eat.

To make hummus, we blended tender chickpeas with a splash of lemon juice and tahini, a creamy sesame paste. As they watched the transformation of simple ingredients into a smooth and delectable spread, their curiosity was piqued.

Next, we laid out an array of colorful vegetables—crisp lettuce, sweet bell peppers, crunchy cucumbers, and ripe avocados. Each vegetable was carefully chosen for its nutrition and the spectrum of tastes and textures it added to the wraps.

As we assembled the Veggie Wraps, I explained how the chickpeas in hummus were a fantastic source of protein, essential for growing bodies, and how the vegetables provided a rainbow of vitamins and minerals, fueling them with vitality.

With excitement and trepidation, they took their first bite, and their faces transformed from uncertainty to delight. The creamy hummus embraced the fresh vegetables, creating a harmonious dance of flavors that danced on their taste buds.

From that moment on, Veggie Wraps with Hummus became a symbol of culinary adventure and a newfound appreciation for trying new things. It was a meal that encouraged them to embrace flavors beyond their comfort zone and discover the joy of exploration in the kitchen.

This chapter celebrates the magic of culinary exploration and the delight of savoring the unexpected. As you and your young chefs prepare Veggie Wraps with Hummus together, may you find joy in discovering new flavors, and may the kitchen be a canvas for creativity and adventure. Bon appétit!

Veggie Wraps with Hummus:

Ingredients:
- Whole-grain or spinach tortilla wraps
- Hummus (store-bought or homemade)
- Assorted fresh vegetables (e.g., lettuce, carrots, cucumbers, bell peppers, etc.)

Instructions:

1. Wash and prepare the fresh vegetables. Cut them into thin strips or slices, making them easier to wrap.

2. Lay out one whole-grain or spinach tortilla wrap on a clean surface.

3. Spread a generous amount of hummus evenly across the entire surface of the tortilla.

4. Place the fresh vegetable strips in the center of the tortilla, leaving some space around the edges.

5. Gently fold one side of the tortilla over the veggies.

6. Fold in the edges of the tortilla.

7. Continue rolling the tortilla until you have a tight and compact wrap.

8. Slice the veggie wrap diagonally in the middle for easier handling.

9. Repeat the process for additional wraps.

10. Serve the veggie wraps with hummus and enjoy!

**Inspire young chefs to see the endless possibilities in combining ingredients and flavors, just like the colorful and delightful veggie wraps they create. Happy wrapping and exploring new flavors!

5

Chicken and Vegetable Stir-Fry

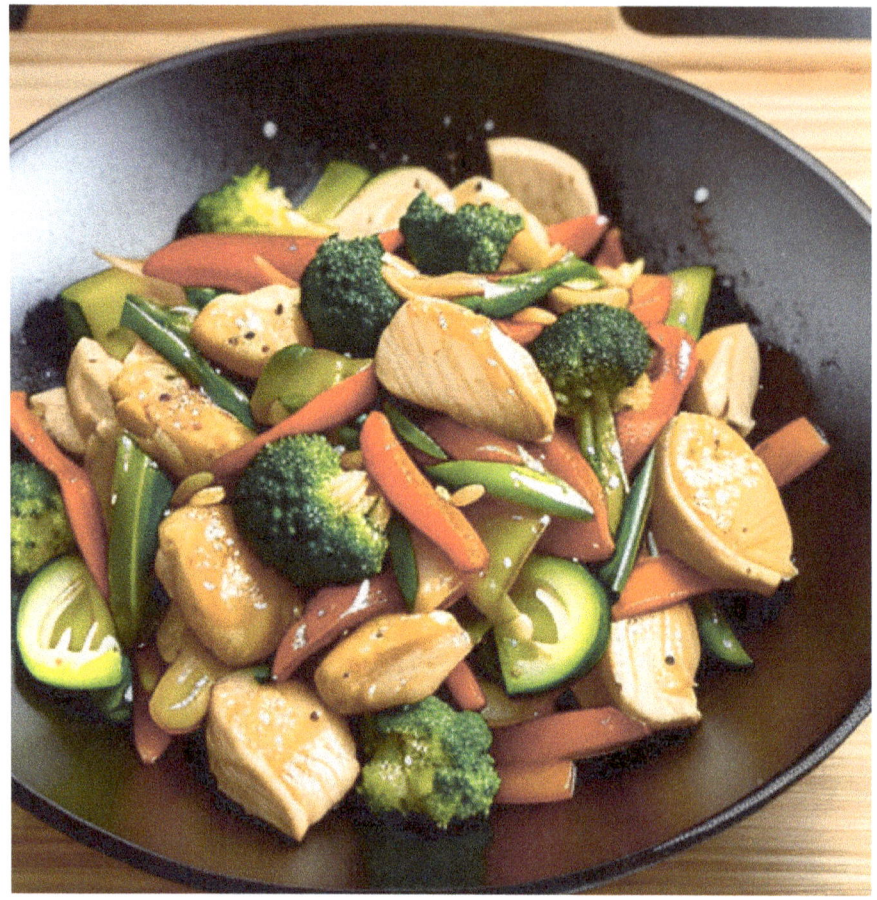

Chicken and Vegetable Stir-Fry

"*In every stir-fry, you have the power to balance flavors and create harmony. Embrace the sizzle and dance of colors, and watch your confidence soar in the kitchen!*"
- **Divine Family Unit**

In our kitchen, there's a dish that never fails to ignite a spark of excitement in my sons' eyes—Chicken and Vegetable Stir-Fry. This meal has become a symbol of togetherness and joy, celebrating the thrill of anticipation as we gather around the dinner table.

It all began on a bustling weeknight when time was scarce, but the desire for a wholesome and flavorful meal was strong. As we set to work, I introduced them to the stars of our stir-fry—tender pieces of chicken, marinated in a blend of soy sauce, ginger, and garlic, creating a symphony of savory goodness.

We chopped an array of colorful vegetables—crisp bell peppers, vibrant broccoli florets, and sweet snow peas, each selected for its vibrant colors and nutrients that would nourish their growing bodies.

The sizzle of the stir-fry filled the kitchen, and the aroma was simply irresistible. Their anticipation mounted with each passing second, and they eagerly peeked into the wok, their senses filled with the promise of a delicious meal.

As we sat down to eat, their excitement reached its peak. They savored every bite, delighting in the medley of flavors and textures that danced on their palates. The tender chicken and crisp vegetables were a symphony of tastes, celebrating the harmony of fresh ingredients coming together.

From that moment on, Chicken and Vegetable Stir-Fry became a cherished dinner ritual, a meal that brought our family together around the table, sharing stories and laughter as we savored the delicious feast.

This chapter celebrates the joy of family gatherings and the pleasure of enjoying a meal made with love and enthusiasm. As you and your young chefs prepare Chicken and Vegetable Stir-Fry together, may you embrace the spirit of togetherness and the anticipation of savoring each moment shared around the dinner table. Bon appétit!

Chicken and Vegetable Stir-Fry:

Ingredients:

- 1 boneless, skinless chicken breast (sliced into thin strips)
- 2 cups mixed vegetables (e.g., broccoli, bell peppers, carrots, snap peas, etc.)
- 2 tablespoons vegetable oil
- 2 tablespoons soy sauce
- 1 tablespoon honey (optional, for a touch of sweetness)
- 1 teaspoon minced garlic
- 1/2 teaspoon grated ginger (optional, for added flavor)
- Cooked rice or noodles (to serve)

Instructions:

1. Wash and prepare the vegetables. Cut them into bite-sized pieces for easy cooking.

2. In a small bowl, mix soy sauce, honey (if using), minced garlic, and grated ginger to create the stir-fry sauce. Set it aside.

3. Heat 1 tablespoon of vegetable oil in a large skillet or wok over medium-high heat.

4. Add the sliced chicken to the skillet and cook until it's no longer pink and cooked through. Remove the cooked chicken from the skillet and set it aside.

5. In the same skillet, add another tablespoon of vegetable oil and then the mixed vegetables. Stir-fry the vegetables for 3-4 minutes or until they become tender-crisp.

6. Return the cooked chicken to the skillet with the vegetables.

7. Pour the stir-fry sauce over the chicken and vegetables. Toss everything together to coat the ingredients evenly with the sauce.

8. Cook for another 1-2 minutes until the sauce thickens slightly and coats the chicken and vegetables.

9. Remove the skillet from the heat.

10. Serve the chicken and vegetable stir-fry over cooked rice or noodles.

**Encourage young chefs to enjoy the process of balancing flavors and textures, just like the beautiful dance of colors in their stir-fry creations. Happy stir-frying and culinary adventures!

6

Peanut Butter and Banana Sandwich on Whole-Grain Bread

PEANUT BUTTER AND BANANA SANDWICH ON WHOLE-GRAIN BREAD

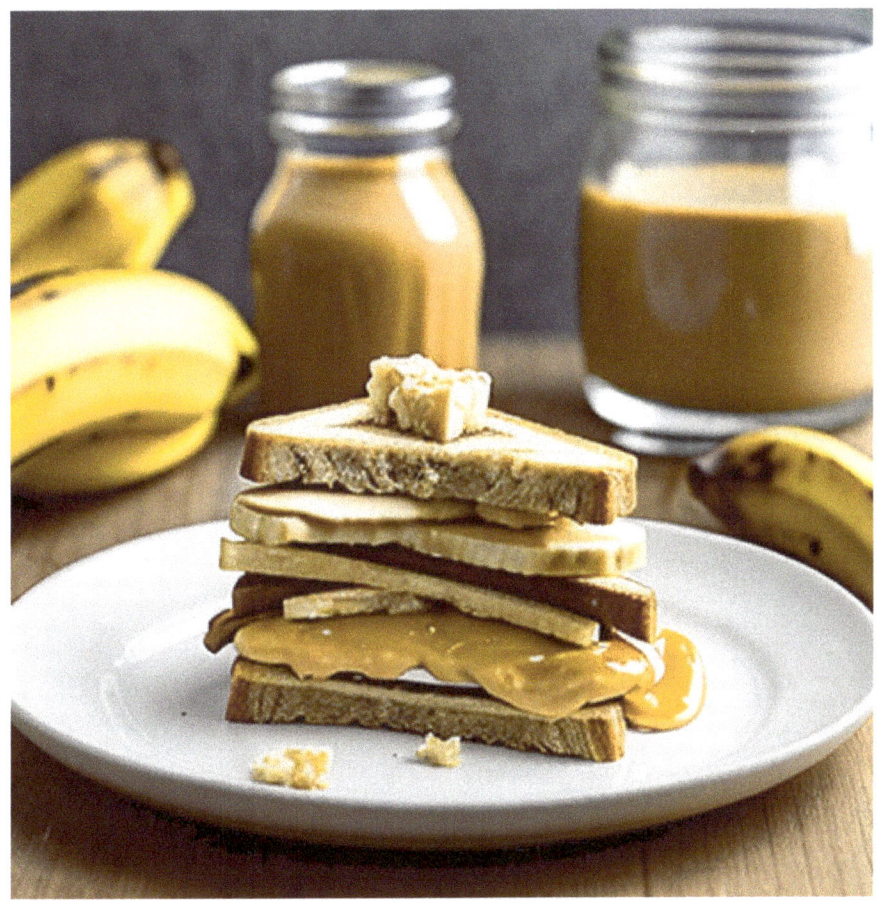

Peanut Butter and Banana Sandwich on Whole-Grain Bread

"*In every sandwich, you hold the power to create a delightful fusion of flavors. Embrace the simplicity, and with each bite, feel the joy of your culinary creation!*" - Divine Family Unit

In our culinary journey, there was a time when my sons thought I was weaving a joke as I unveiled a seemingly peculiar combination—Peanut Butter and Banana Sandwich on Whole-Grain Bread. Little did they know that this delightful sandwich would soon become a beloved staple, evoking smiles and satisfaction with every bite.

One sunny afternoon, I decided to introduce them to a timeless classic—a peanut butter and banana sandwich. As I spread creamy peanut butter on slices of hearty whole-grain bread, their curiosity was piqued. The combination of nutty richness and sweet, ripe bananas seemed unconventional, but I assured them it was a delightful pairing.

The whole-grain bread was carefully chosen for its nutritional value, providing fiber and essential nutrients to keep their bodies strong and energized. I explained how peanut butter, a great source of protein and healthy fats, would keep their tummies full and their hearts happy.

As they took their first bite, their faces transformed from skepticism to sheer joy. The creaminess of the peanut butter harmonized with the sweet banana, creating a delectable medley of flavors that they couldn't resist.

From that moment on, the Peanut Butter and Banana Sandwich on Whole-Grain Bread became a lunchtime favorite. It was a meal they could prepare with ease and enjoy with enthusiasm, a delightful combination that brought smiles and satisfaction to their young hearts.

This chapter celebrates the magic of unexpected pairings and the joy of discovering new tastes. As you and your young chefs prepare this delightful sandwich together, may you savor the simplicity and the joy it brings, a culinary union that transcends the ordinary and becomes an extraordinary delight. Bon appétit!

Peanut Butter and Banana Sandwich on Whole-Grain Bread:

Ingredients:
  - 2 slices of whole-grain bread
  - 2 tablespoons peanut butter (smooth or crunchy)
  - 1 ripe banana, sliced

PEANUT BUTTER AND BANANA SANDWICH ON WHOLE-GRAIN BREAD

Instructions:

1. Lay out the two slices of whole-grain bread on a clean surface.

2. Using a butter knife or spoon, spread the peanut butter on one side of each bread slice.

3. Peel the ripe banana and slice it into thin rounds.

4. Arrange the banana slices on top of the peanut butter spread on one of the bread slices.

5. Carefully place the other bread slice with the peanut butter spread on top of the banana slices to create a sandwich.

6. Gently press the sandwich together to make sure it sticks together.

7. If you prefer, you can cut the sandwich diagonally to create two triangles or straight across for two rectangles.

8. Your peanut butter and banana sandwich on whole-grain bread is ready to enjoy!

**Inspire young chefs to appreciate the joy of creating simple and delicious dishes like the peanut butter and banana sandwich. Cooking is about enjoying the process and the satisfying result. Happy sandwich-making and savoring the flavors!

7

Fruit Salad with a Drizzle of Honey

FRUIT SALAD WITH A DRIZZLE OF HONEY

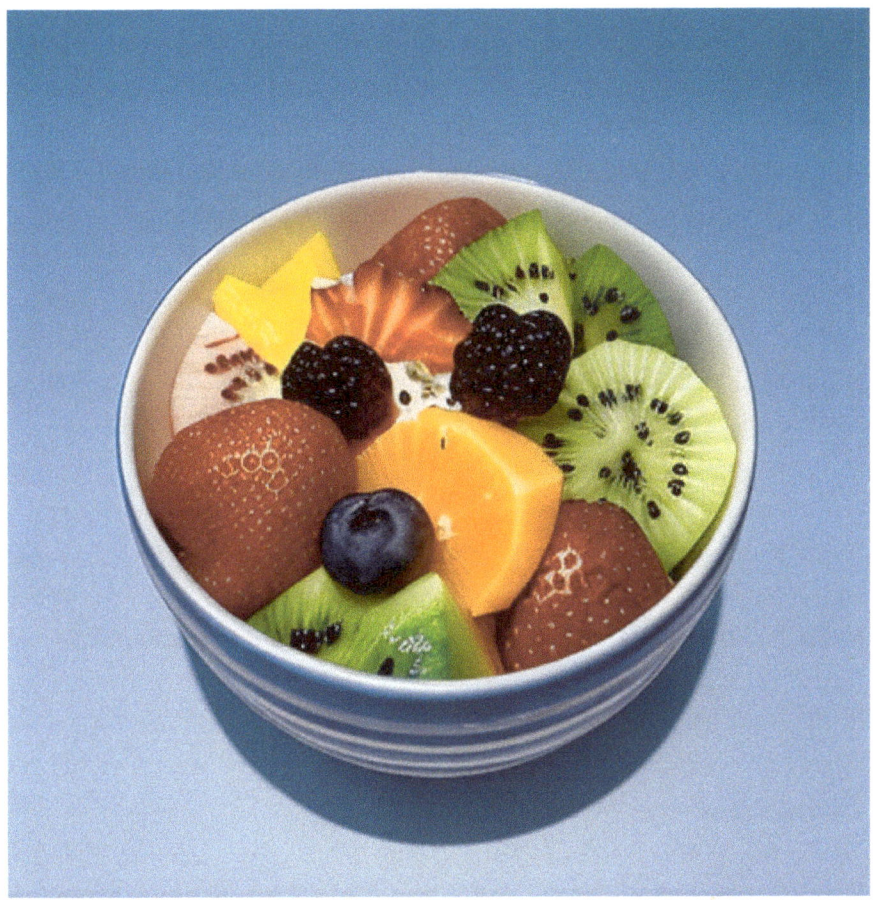

Fruit Salad with a Drizzle of Honey

"*In every fruit salad, you have the power to blend colors and flavors in perfect harmony. Embrace the vibrant variety, and watch your creativity shine in every delicious bite!*"
- Papa True Ju

In our home, there's a meal that never fails to summon a flurry of excitement—the Fruit Salad with a Drizzle of Honey. This vibrant and refreshing creation charges my sons with positive energy, and they can't resist racing to the kitchen table when they catch a glimpse of its colorful allure.

One sunny morning, as the day began to unfold, I decided to surprise my sons with a delightful fruit salad. As they gathered around the kitchen, their eyes widened with anticipation as they saw an array of fruits—juicy watermelon, succulent strawberries, sweet blueberries, and tangy oranges, each chosen for its burst of flavor and nutritional goodness.

The fruit salad was a burst of colors—a feast for the eyes and the senses. I explained that the fruits were not only rich in vitamins and antioxidants but also packed with natural sugars that would provide them with a refreshing burst of energy to start their day.

But the magic didn't end there. A drizzle of honey was the final touch—a touch of golden sweetness that brought out the natural flavors of the fruits and added a hint of decadence to the salad. I shared with them how honey was not only a natural sweetener but also had various health benefits.

As they took their first spoonfuls, a chorus of "Mmm!" and "Yum!" filled the kitchen. Their faces lit up with joy as they savored the medley of flavors, discovering new combinations with each bite.

From that moment on, the Fruit Salad with a Drizzle of Honey became a breakfast favorite. It was a quick and easy meal they could prepare themselves, infusing their mornings with a burst of positive energy and the promise of a day filled with vitality.

This chapter celebrates the beauty of simplicity and the joy of embracing nature's bounty. As you and your young chefs prepare this vibrant fruit salad together, may you relish the magic of colors and flavors, and may it fuel your hearts and souls with the positive energy to seize each day with zest. Bon appétit!

Fruit Salad with a Drizzle of Honey:

FRUIT SALAD WITH A DRIZZLE OF HONEY

Ingredients:

- Assorted fresh fruits (e.g., strawberries, blueberries, grapes, kiwi, pineapple, etc.)
- 1-2 tablespoons honey (or to taste)

Instructions:

1. Wash and prepare the fresh fruits. Peel, slice, and cut them into bite-sized pieces as needed.

2. Add the assorted fresh fruits to a mixing bowl.

3. Drizzle 1-2 tablespoons of honey over the fruits in the bowl.

4. Gently toss the fruits with the honey, ensuring that the honey coats each fruit piece.

5. Taste the fruit salad and adjust the sweetness by adding more honey if desired.

6. Serve the fruit salad in individual bowls or plates.

**Encourage young chefs to enjoy the artistry of creating colorful and flavorful fruit salads, making each bite a delightful experience. Cooking is a canvas for creativity, and fruit salads are a perfect place to showcase that creativity. Happy fruit salad making and artistic expression!

8

Turkey and Cheese Roll-Ups

TURKEY AND CHEESE ROLL-UPS

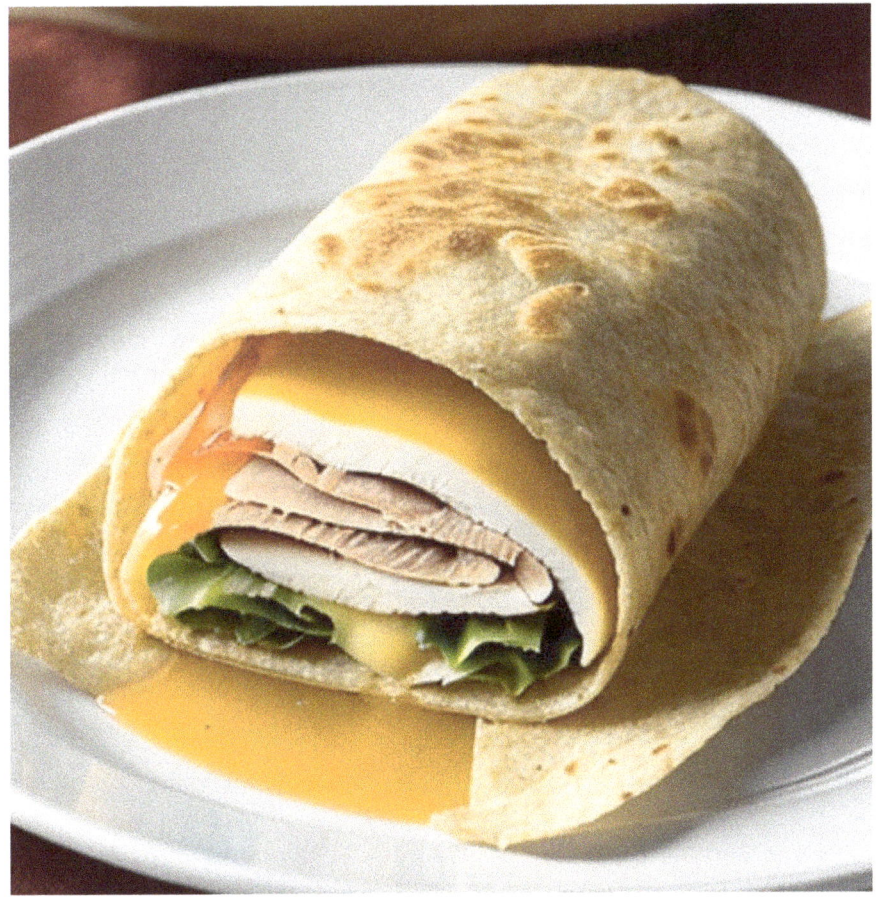

Turkey and Cheese Roll-Up

"*In every roll-up, you have the power to wrap joy and goodness. Embrace the simplicity, and with each bite, feel the delight of your culinary creation!*" - *Unknown*

In our culinary journey, there's a quick meal that never fails to light up my sons' faces with excitement—the Turkey and Cheese Roll-Ups. This delightful creation has become their go-to lunchtime favorite, a simple dish that always brings smiles and happiness.

One bustling afternoon, as we gathered in the kitchen, my sons caught a glimpse of the ingredients laid out before them—thin slices of savory turkey, a medley of creamy cheeses, and crisp lettuce leaves, all carefully chosen for their complementary flavors and textures.

As I showed them how to roll the turkey slices around the cheese and lettuce, their eyes sparkled with anticipation. I explained that the turkey provided a great source of lean protein, essential for their active bodies, while the cheese added a burst of creaminess that made every bite a delight.

With excitement, they rolled up their creations, eagerly tasting each bite as they assembled their turkey and cheese masterpieces. Their smiles grew wider with every mouthful, and they marveled at how such a simple meal could bring them so much joy.

From that moment on, the Turkey and Cheese Roll-Ups became a lunchtime tradition, a meal they could prepare with ease and enthusiasm. Whether it was for a quick bite before heading out to play or a satisfying lunch at home, the roll-ups never failed to make them happy.

This chapter celebrates the beauty of simplicity and the joy of creating delicious meals with just a few ingredients. As you and your young chefs prepare these delightful roll-ups together, may you savor the joy of assembling each bite and the happiness that comes from sharing a meal made with love. Bon appétit!

Turkey and Cheese Roll-Ups:

Ingredients:
- Sliced turkey (deli turkey or leftover roasted turkey)
- Sliced cheese (cheddar, Swiss, or your favorite cheese)
- Whole-grain tortilla or flatbread

Instructions:

TURKEY AND CHEESE ROLL-UPS

1. Lay out a whole-grain tortilla or flatbread on a clean surface.

2. Place a few slices of turkey evenly on the tortilla, leaving some space around the edges.

3. Lay a slice of cheese on top of the turkey.

4. Carefully roll the tortilla from one end to create a tight and compact roll-up.

5. If the tortilla isn't sticking together, you can use a thin layer of hummus or cream cheese along the edge to seal it.

6. Slice the roll-up into bite-sized pinwheels or simply serve it as a whole roll.

7. You can use a toothpick to secure the pinwheels if desired.

8. Your turkey and cheese roll-ups are ready to enjoy!

**Inspire young chefs to find joy in creating simple yet delicious meals like turkey and cheese roll-ups. The process of rolling and slicing can be fun and rewarding. Happy rolling and savoring the flavors!

9

Avocado Toast with a Sprinkle of Sesame Seeds

AVOCADO TOAST WITH A SPRINKLE OF SESAME SEEDS

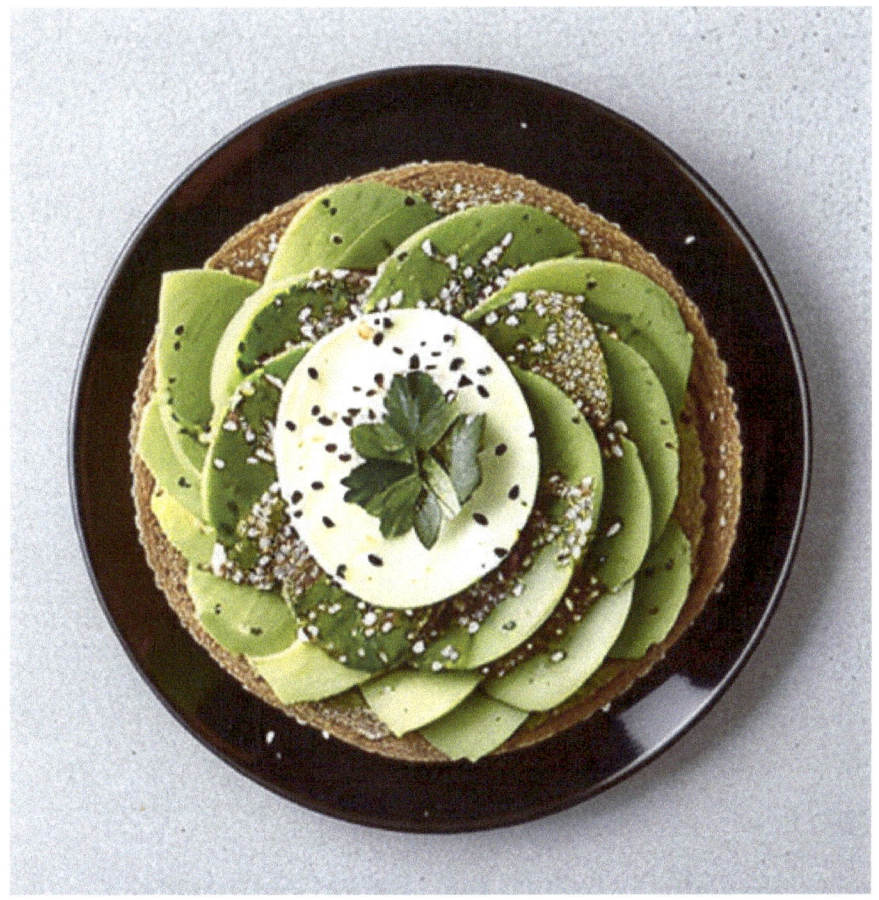

Avocado Toast with a Sprinkle of Sesame Seeds

"*In every toast, you have the power to spread joy and goodness. Embrace the simplicity, and with every bite, feel the magic of your culinary creation!*" - Papa True Ju

In our kitchen, there's a quick meal that never fails to light up my sons' faces with joy—the Avocado Toast with a Sprinkle of Sesame Seeds. This delightful creation has become a cherished favorite, a simple dish that always brings smiles and happiness to our table.

One sunny morning, as the day began to unfold, my sons eagerly gathered around the kitchen counter, their eyes alight with anticipation. They knew that the ingredients before them held the promise of a satisfying and nutritious breakfast.

Ripe avocados, creamy and buttery, were carefully mashed, ready to be spread atop slices of hearty whole-grain toast. I explained how avocados were a treasure trove of healthy fats, essential for their growing bodies, and how the whole-grain toast added a delightful crunch while providing fiber and vital nutrients.

As they carefully arranged the avocado on the toast, a sprinkle of sesame seeds was the finishing touch, adding a nutty and toasty flavor that elevated the dish to a new level of deliciousness. I shared with them the nutritional benefits of sesame seeds, rich in vitamins and minerals that would nourish their minds and bodies.

With excitement, they took their first bites, savoring the creamy avocado mingling with the satisfying crunch of the toast. The sesame seeds added a delightful surprise, delighting their taste buds with every mouthful.

From that moment on, Avocado Toast with a Sprinkle of Sesame Seeds became a breakfast ritual, a meal they could prepare with ease and enthusiasm. Whether it was a leisurely weekend breakfast or a quick bite before school, the avocado toast always brought a smile to their faces.

This chapter celebrates the beauty of simple pleasures and the joy of discovering new flavors. As you and your young chefs prepare this delightful avocado toast together, may you savor the satisfaction of creating a wholesome and delicious meal and the happiness that comes from sharing it with loved ones. Bon appétit!

Avocado Toast with a Sprinkle of Sesame Seeds:

AVOCADO TOAST WITH A SPRINKLE OF SESAME SEEDS

Ingredients:
- 1 ripe avocado
- 2 slices of whole-grain bread (toasted)
- Sprinkle of sesame seeds
- Salt and pepper to taste

Instructions:

1. Cut the ripe avocado in half and remove the pit.

2. Scoop the avocado flesh into a bowl.

3. Mash the avocado with a fork until it reaches your desired consistency (smooth or slightly chunky).

4. Add a pinch of salt and pepper to the mashed avocado, and mix it in for extra flavor.

5. Toast two slices of whole-grain bread until they are lightly browned and crispy.

6. Spread the mashed avocado evenly on each slice of toasted bread.

7. Sprinkle a generous amount of sesame seeds over the avocado spread on both slices of toast.

8. Your avocado toast with a sprinkle of sesame seeds is now ready to enjoy!

**Encourage young chefs to appreciate the simplicity and versatility of avocado toast and to embrace the joy of creating delicious and nutritious meals. Happy toasting and savoring the magic of flavors!

10

Tuna Salad Lettuce Wraps

TUNA SALAD LETTUCE WRAPS

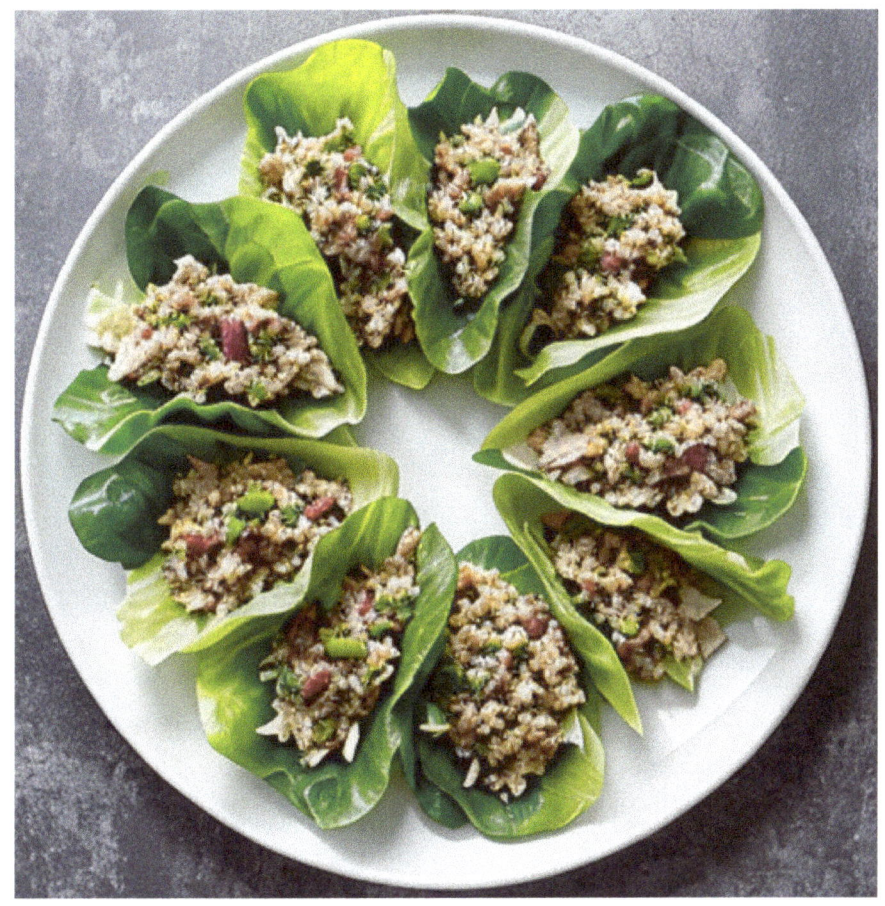

Tuna Salad Lettuce Wraps

"*In every wrap, you hold the power to create a masterpiece of flavor and balance. Embrace the journey, and with every bite, feel the pride of your culinary creation!*" - *Coach Rae*

In our culinary journey, there's a quick meal that gives my sons the extra boost they need for their sports training—the Tuna Salad Lettuce Wraps. This energizing and delicious dish has become their go-to choice, fueling their active bodies with the power of wholesome ingredients.

On a sunny day, as they prepared for their sports training, I knew they needed a meal that would provide sustained energy and nourishment. Together, we crafted the Tuna Salad Lettuce Wraps—a delightful fusion of fresh and vibrant flavors.

Chunks of flavorful tuna were mixed with crisp celery, crunchy bell peppers, and juicy cherry tomatoes. I explained that the tuna was an excellent source of lean protein, essential for their muscle development and endurance, while the vegetables added a burst of vitamins and antioxidants to keep them going strong.

We lovingly folded the tuna salad into large, tender lettuce leaves, creating a delightful wrap that was not only nutritious but also refreshing. I shared with them the benefits of using lettuce as a wrap, providing a lighter and carb-conscious alternative to traditional bread.

With excitement, they bit into their lettuce wraps, savoring the medley of flavors and textures. The tuna salad provided the protein punch they needed, while the vegetables offered a delightful crunch, invigorating their taste buds and boosting their spirits.

From that moment on, Tuna Salad Lettuce Wraps became their sports training fuel, a quick and satisfying meal that powered them through their activities with enthusiasm.

This chapter celebrates the magic of food as fuel and the joy of creating nourishing meals that support our young athletes. As you and your young chefs prepare these energizing lettuce wraps together, may you savor the sense of vitality they provide and the happiness that comes from nourishing your bodies for the adventures that lie ahead. Bon appétit!

Tuna Salad Lettuce Wraps:

Ingredients:

TUNA SALAD LETTUCE WRAPS

- 1 can tuna (in water or oil, drained)
- 2 tablespoons mayonnaise (or Greek yogurt for a lighter option)
- 1 tablespoon diced celery
- 1 tablespoon diced red onion
- Salt and pepper to taste
- Large lettuce leaves (e.g., romaine or iceberg)

Instructions:

1. In a bowl, mix the drained tuna, mayonnaise (or Greek yogurt), diced celery, and diced red onion.

2. Add a pinch of salt and pepper to taste. Mix everything until well combined.

3. Wash and dry large lettuce leaves. Pat them gently with a paper towel to remove excess moisture.

4. Place a spoonful of the tuna salad mixture onto the center of each lettuce leaf.

5. Carefully fold the sides of the lettuce leaf over the tuna mixture to create a wrap.

6. Secure the wrap with a toothpick if needed.

7. Repeat the process for additional wraps.

8. Your tuna salad lettuce wraps are ready to enjoy!

**Encourage young chefs to take pride in their creations and to enjoy the process of balancing flavors and textures in their tuna salad lettuce wraps. Cooking is a journey of discovery and deliciousness. Happy wrapping and culinary adventure!

11

Quinoa Salad with Veggies and Feta Cheese

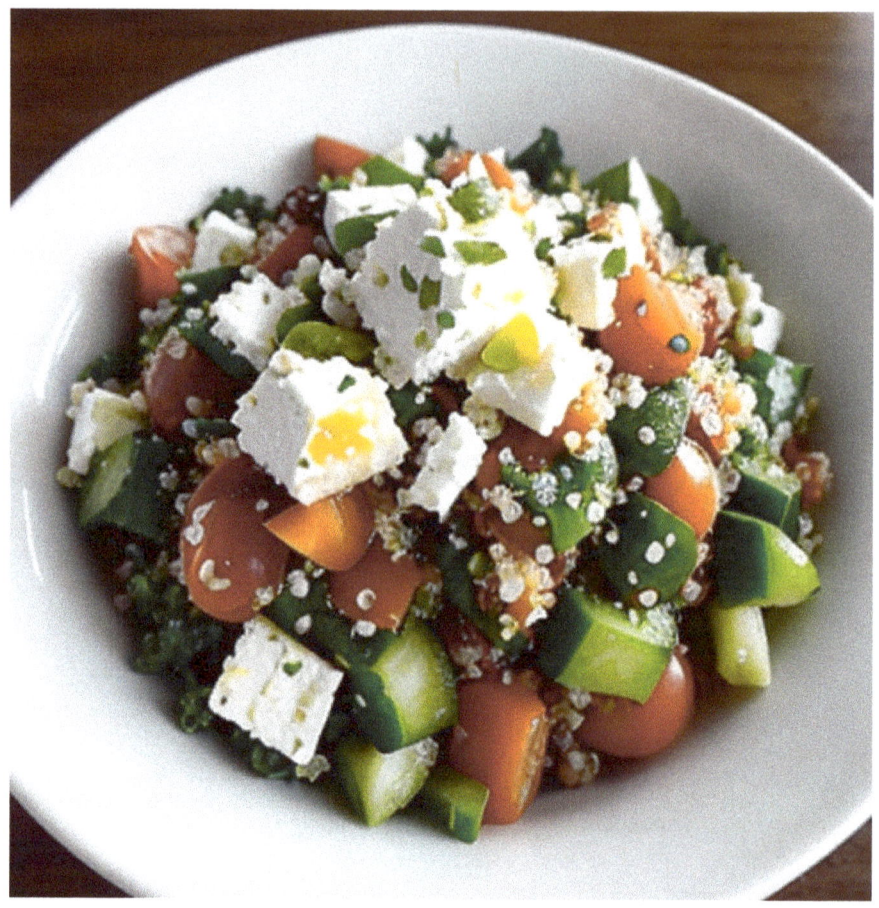

Quinoa Salad with Veggies and Feta Cheese

"*In every salad, you have the power to mix colors and textures like a true artist. Embrace the canvas of flavors, and with every bite, feel the pride of your culinary creation!*" - Unknown

In our kitchen, there's a quick meal that fills my sons' tummies and warms their hearts—the Quinoa Salad with Veggies and Feta Cheese. This wholesome and flavorful dish has become a cherished favorite, a testament to their evolving taste buds and the joy of trying new flavors.

One sunny afternoon, as we set out to create a nutritious and delicious salad, my sons weren't quite sure about the feta cheese that lay before them. But they were eager to embrace the adventure and explore the world of flavors that awaited them.

We cooked a fluffy batch of protein-rich quinoa, setting the foundation for the salad. I explained how quinoa was a nutritional powerhouse, providing a complete protein source, essential for their growing bodies.

We chopped an array of colorful vegetables—crisp cucumbers, juicy cherry tomatoes, and tangy red onions, each selected for its vibrant colors and nutrients that would nourish their bodies and delight their taste buds.

With curiosity and trepidation, they tasted a morsel of feta cheese. To their surprise, the salty and creamy flavors danced on their palates, adding a delightful twist to the salad.

As we tossed the quinoa with the vegetables and feta cheese, a medley of colors and textures came together, forming a vibrant and satisfying salad. The feta cheese harmonized with the fresh vegetables, creating a taste experience they had grown to love.

From that moment on, the Quinoa Salad with Veggies and Feta Cheese became a celebrated lunchtime favorite, a quick and nutritious meal that filled their tummies and warmed their hearts.

This chapter celebrates the joy of embracing new flavors and the pleasure of discovering culinary delights. As you and your young chefs prepare this vibrant quinoa salad together, may you savor the adventure of exploring new tastes and the happiness that comes from nourishing your bodies with wholesome and delightful meals. Bon appétit!

Quinoa Salad with Veggies and Feta Cheese:

Ingredients:
- 1 cup cooked quinoa
- Assorted vegetables (e.g., cherry tomatoes, cucumber, bell peppers, red onion, etc.)
- 1/4 cup crumbled feta cheese
- Fresh herbs (e.g., parsley, basil, or cilantro) for added flavor (optional)

Instructions:

1. Cook the quinoa according to the package instructions. Let it cool completely before making the salad.

2. Wash and prepare the vegetables. Cut them into small, bite-sized pieces.

3. In a large mixing bowl, combine the cooked quinoa, assorted vegetables, and crumbled feta cheese.

4. If you like, you can also add some fresh herbs, like parsley, basil, or cilantro, for an extra burst of flavor.

5. Gently toss all the ingredients together until they are well-mixed.

6. Taste the quinoa salad and adjust the seasoning if needed by adding a pinch of salt and pepper.

7. Your quinoa salad with veggies and feta cheese is ready to serve!

**Inspire young chefs to see their quinoa salad as a work of art, where they can combine colors, textures, and flavors to create a beautiful and nutritious dish. Cooking is an opportunity to express creativity and enjoy delicious outcomes. Happy salad-making and artistic expression!

12

Veggie Sushi Rolls

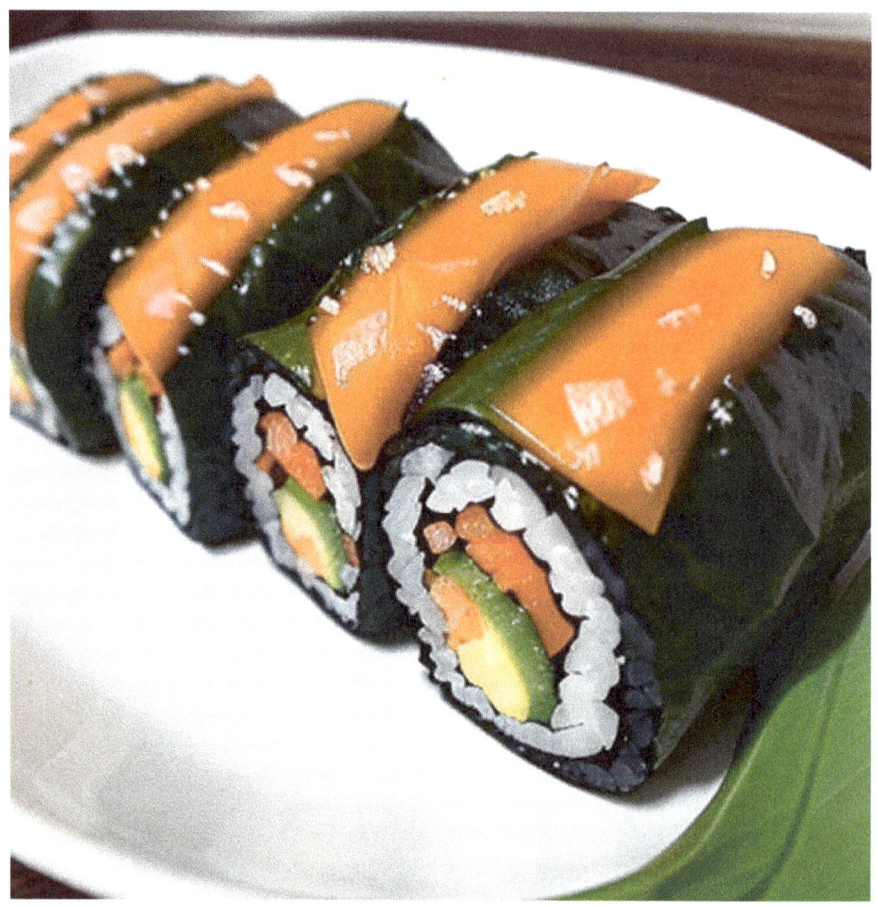

Veggie Sushi Rolls

"*In every sushi roll, you hold the power to roll perfection and create a taste of Japan. Embrace the art of precision, and with every bite, feel the pride of your culinary creation!*"
- Divine Family Unit

In our culinary journey, there's a tale of inspiration that led my sons to embrace the world of sushi—the Veggie Sushi Rolls. Their mother, a lover of traditional fish-based sushi rolls, sparked their curiosity with her enthusiasm, motivating them to explore a delightful and wholesome alternative.

As they watched their mother savor the flavors of traditional sushi, their interest grew. However, being young adventurers with evolving tastes, they were unsure about raw fish. Undeterred, their mother introduced them to Veggie Sushi Rolls—a delightful fusion of vibrant vegetables and seasoned rice.

Together, we gathered an array of fresh and colorful vegetables—crisp cucumbers, ripe avocados, and sweet carrots—each chosen for its delectable taste and nutritional goodness.

With curiosity and excitement, they rolled the vegetables into tender nori seaweed sheets, along with seasoned sushi rice. As they assembled their sushi rolls, they marveled at the colors and textures that came together, eager to taste the creation they had crafted with their own hands.

With a dash of soy sauce and a dollop of wasabi, they took their first bites, their taste buds dancing with delight. The Veggie Sushi Rolls provided a medley of flavors, a wholesome and satisfying alternative to traditional sushi.

From that moment on, Veggie Sushi Rolls became a cherished favorite, a quick and fun meal they could prepare themselves. They not only enjoyed the vibrant flavors but also felt a sense of accomplishment in creating something as beautiful and delicious as their mother's beloved sushi.

This chapter celebrates the joy of exploration and the magic of culinary creativity. As you and your young chefs prepare these delightful Veggie Sushi Rolls together, may you savor the inspiration that led them on this culinary adventure and the happiness that comes from embracing wholesome and delicious alternatives. Bon appétit!

Veggie Sushi Rolls:

Ingredients:

- Sushi rice (cooked and seasoned with rice vinegar, sugar, and salt)
- Nori seaweed sheets
- Assorted vegetables (e.g., cucumber, avocado, carrots, bell peppers, etc.)
- Soy sauce and pickled ginger for dipping (optional)

Instructions:

1. Prepare the sushi rice according to the package instructions. Once cooked, let it cool to room temperature and season it with a mixture of rice vinegar, sugar, and salt for added flavor.

2. Wash and prepare the vegetables. Cut them into thin strips or slices.

3. Lay a bamboo sushi rolling mat on a clean surface. If you don't have a bamboo mat, you can use plastic wrap as a substitute.

4. Place a sheet of nori seaweed on the bamboo mat with the shiny side facing down.

5. Wet your fingers to prevent sticking and spread a thin layer of sushi rice evenly over the nori, leaving about 1 inch of the top edge uncovered.

6. Arrange the assorted vegetable strips or slices horizontally across the rice, slightly below the center of the nori sheet.

7. Carefully lift the bamboo mat from the bottom edge and start rolling the nori sheet and rice around the vegetables. Use gentle pressure to create a tight roll.

8. Once you reach the uncovered edge of the nori, moisten it slightly with water to help seal the roll.

9. Continue rolling until the entire sheet is wrapped around the rice and

vegetables.

10. Use a sharp knife to slice the sushi roll into bite-sized pieces. Wet the knife between cuts to avoid sticking.

11. Arrange the sushi rolls on a plate and serve with soy sauce and pickled ginger for dipping, if desired.

**Inspire young chefs to appreciate the precision and artistry of making sushi rolls, and to take pride in their culinary creations. Sushi-making can be a fun and rewarding experience in the kitchen. Happy rolling and enjoying the taste of Japan!

13

Baked Sweet Potato Fries

BAKED SWEET POTATO FRIES

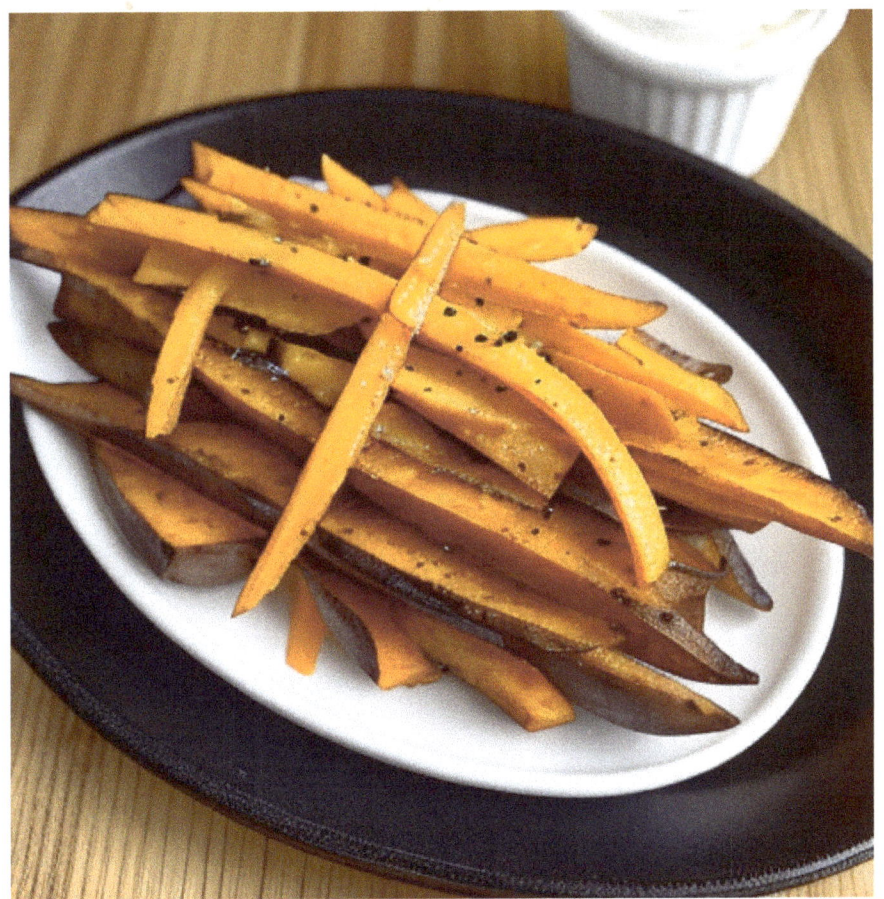

Baked Sweet Potato Fries

"*In every sweet potato fry, you have the power to bake goodness and savor the feeling of victory. Embrace the magic of simple pleasures, and with every bite, taste the joy of your culinary creation!*" - Papa True Ju

In our kitchen, there's a tale of love for all things fries that led my sons to embark on a healthy and flavorful adventure—the Baked Sweet Potato Fries. Their fondness for fries motivated them to explore a wholesome but delicious alternative, creating a meal that satisfied both their taste buds and their desire for nutritious options.

With fries being a favorite indulgence, we set out to create a healthier version that would still delight their palates. Together, we chose sweet potatoes, vibrant and nutrient-rich, as the star ingredient.

As we sliced the sweet potatoes into slender strips, their cheerful orange hues filled the kitchen with warmth. I explained how sweet potatoes were packed with vitamins and antioxidants, providing a burst of flavor and nourishment to their growing bodies.

To ensure a crispy and flavorful outcome, we drizzled the sweet potato strips with a dash of olive oil, sprinkled with a pinch of salt, and a hint of aromatic herbs. As they placed the seasoned fries on a baking tray, their excitement grew, eager to taste the result of their culinary efforts.

As the aroma of baking sweet potatoes filled the air, they could hardly contain their anticipation. When the fries emerged from the oven, crispy and golden, their eyes sparkled with delight.

With the first bite, their taste buds were met with a delightful contrast of crispy exterior and tender interior. The sweet potatoes offered a natural sweetness that was both comforting and nutritious, earning a special place in their hearts as a beloved alternative to traditional fries.

From that moment on, Baked Sweet Potato Fries became a cherished go-to snack, a quick and delicious meal they could prepare anytime. It was a culinary triumph, proving that healthy choices could be just as delightful and satisfying as their favorite indulgences.

This chapter celebrates the joy of healthy alternatives and the magic of creating flavorsome meals that nourish the body and delight the senses. As you and your young chefs prepare these delightful Baked Sweet Potato Fries together, may you savor the journey of discovery and the happiness that comes from making wholesome choices that taste oh-so-good. Bon appétit!

Baked Sweet Potato Fries:

Ingredients:
- 2 medium sweet potatoes
- 2 tablespoons olive oil
- 1/2 teaspoon salt
- 1/4 teaspoon pepper
- Optional seasoning (e.g., paprika, garlic powder, or rosemary)

Instructions:

1. Preheat your oven to 425°F (220°C) and line a baking sheet with parchment paper.

2. Wash and peel the sweet potatoes. Cut them into thin strips to resemble fries.

3. In a large mixing bowl, toss the sweet potato strips with olive oil until they are evenly coated.

4. Sprinkle salt and pepper over the sweet potatoes and toss them again to ensure even seasoning.

5. If you like, you can add a pinch of optional seasoning, such as paprika, garlic powder, or rosemary, for added flavor.

6. Spread the seasoned sweet potato strips in a single layer on the prepared baking sheet.

7. Bake the sweet potato fries in the preheated oven for about 20-25 minutes, or until they are crispy and golden brown, turning them halfway through to ensure even cooking.

8. Once the sweet potato fries are done, remove them from the oven and let them cool slightly.

9. Serve the baked sweet potato fries as a delightful and nutritious side dish.

**Inspire young chefs to find joy in creating simple yet delicious dishes like the baked sweet potato fries, and to savor the satisfaction of preparing a nutritious and tasty treat. Cooking is a delightful experience of victory with every successful dish. Happy baking and savoring the magic of flavors!

14

Spinach and Feta Stuffed Chicken Breast

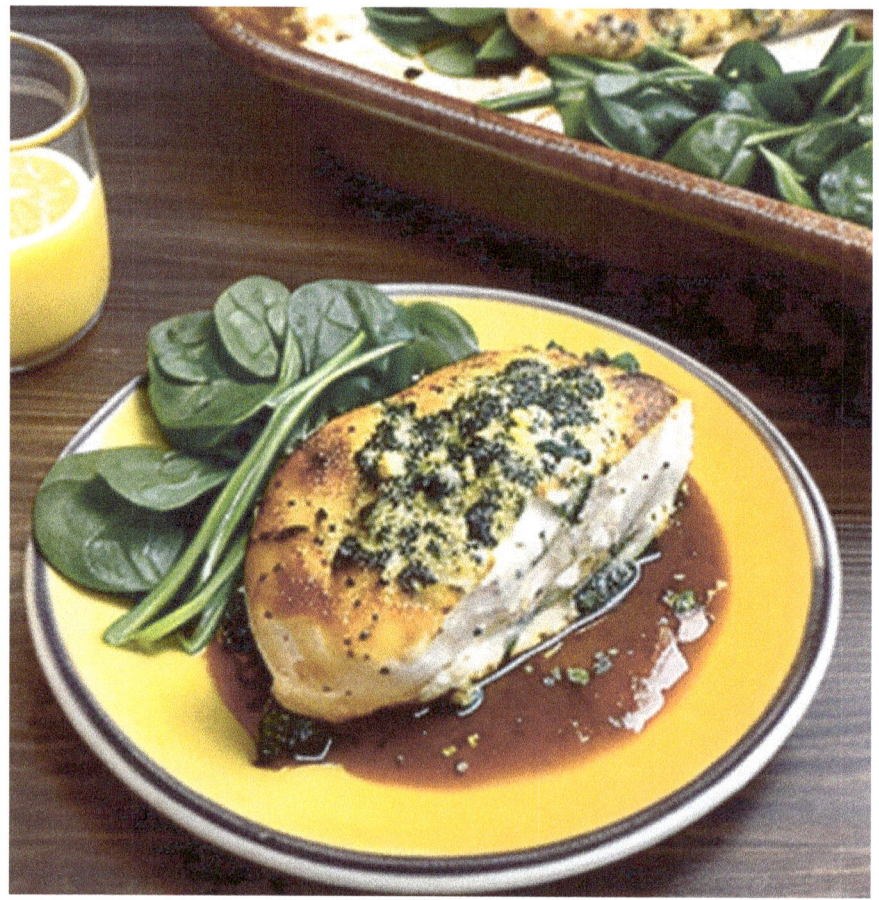

Spinach and Feta Stuffed Chicken Breast

"*In every stuffed chicken breast, you hold the power to create a burst of flavor and a culinary masterpiece. Embrace the art of cooking, and with every bite, feel the pride of your culinary creation!*" - *Divine Family Unit*

In our kitchen, there's a tale of mouthwatering anticipation that led my sons to fall in love with the delightful aroma of Spinach and Feta Stuffed Chicken Breast. This flavorful and wholesome dish has become a family favorite, enticing their taste buds with the promise of a delectable meal.

SPINACH AND FETA STUFFED CHICKEN BREAST

One evening, as we set out to create a meal that celebrated the harmony of flavors, we carefully prepared tender chicken breasts. Together, we concocted a delightful stuffing with a blend of vibrant spinach leaves and creamy feta cheese.

As the chicken breasts were gently folded around the spinach and feta mixture, a delightful aroma filled the air, weaving a tale of savory delights that made their mouths water with excitement.

I explained how spinach was a nutritional powerhouse, rich in vitamins and minerals that would keep their bodies strong and healthy. The feta cheese added a burst of tangy flavor, creating a delightful contrast to the tender chicken.

As the stuffed chicken breasts were baked in the oven, the flavors melded together, creating a symphony of tastes that were both comforting and enticing.

When they took their first bites, their eyes widened with pleasure. The tender chicken embraced the spinach and feta stuffing, creating a harmonious dance of flavors that they couldn't resist.

From that moment on, Spinach and Feta Stuffed Chicken Breast became a cherished dinner staple, a meal that brought our family together around the table, sharing stories and laughter as we savored the delicious feast.

This chapter celebrates the magic of flavors and the joy of coming together with a wholesome and satisfying meal. As you and your young chefs prepare these delightful stuffed chicken breasts together, may you savor the mouthwatering anticipation and the happiness that comes from sharing a delicious and nourishing meal with loved ones. Bon appétit!

Spinach and Feta Stuffed Chicken Breast:

Ingredients:
- 2 boneless, skinless chicken breasts
- 1 cup fresh spinach leaves
- 1/4 cup crumbled feta cheese
- Salt and pepper to taste
- Olive oil or melted butter for brushing

Instructions:

1. Preheat your oven to 375°F (190°C).

2. Using a sharp knife, carefully make a slit in the side of each chicken breast to create a pocket for the stuffing. Be cautious and ask for adult supervision if needed.

3. Season the inside of the chicken breasts with a pinch of salt and pepper.

4. Stuff each chicken breast with fresh spinach leaves and crumbled feta cheese, evenly distributing the filling.

5. Close the opening of the chicken breasts by pressing the edges together.

6. Secure the stuffed chicken breasts with toothpicks, if needed, to ensure the filling stays inside during cooking.

7. Brush the chicken breasts with a little olive oil or melted butter for a golden and moist finish.

8. Place the stuffed chicken breasts in a baking dish.

9. Bake the chicken in the preheated oven for about 25-30 minutes or until the internal temperature reaches 165°F (74°C).

SPINACH AND FETA STUFFED CHICKEN BREAST

10. Once cooked, remove the toothpicks, and let the chicken rest for a few minutes before serving.

11. Slice the stuffed chicken breasts and serve as a delicious and nutritious main course.

**Inspire young chefs to see cooking as an art form, where they can create flavorful and beautiful dishes like spinach and feta stuffed chicken breast. Cooking is an opportunity for artistic expression and culinary mastery. Happy cooking and culinary creativity!

15

Baked Salmon with Lemon and Herbs

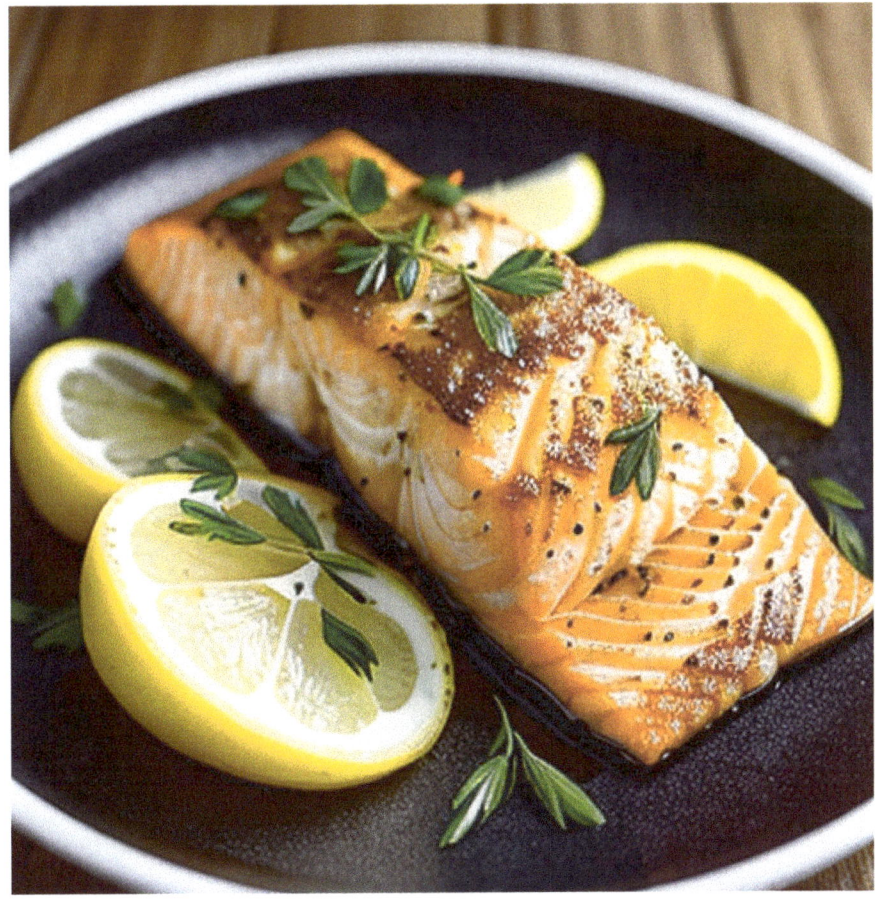

Baked Salmon with Lemon and Herbs

"*In every baked salmon, you hold the power to create a taste of the sea and a feast for the senses. Embrace the flavors of nature, and with every bite, feel the joy of your culinary creation!*" - *Coach Rae*

In our culinary journey, there's a tale of appreciation for wholesome nourishment that led my sons to embrace the goodness of Baked Salmon with Lemon and Herbs. This flavorful and nutritious dish became their secret weapon, providing them with extra focus during study time and sports competitions.

As we embarked on a quest to create a meal that would fuel their minds and bodies, we carefully selected fresh and succulent salmon fillets, known for their abundance of omega-3 fats—a superhero nutrient for brain health and overall well-being.

With excitement, they drizzled the salmon with a burst of fresh lemon juice, infusing it with a zesty and refreshing tang. I explained how lemon not only elevated the flavor of the salmon but also provided a burst of vitamin C, boosting their immune systems.

Next, we adorned the salmon with a medley of fragrant herbs—rosemary, thyme, and parsley, each chosen for their aromatic notes and added nutritional benefits.

As the salmon baked in the oven, their anticipation grew. When it emerged, tender and flaky, the enticing aroma of lemon and herbs filled the air, promising a delectable feast.

When they took their first bites, they marveled at the burst of flavors. The omega-3-rich salmon not only provided brain-boosting goodness but also offered a rich, satisfying taste.

From that moment on, Baked Salmon with Lemon and Herbs became their go-to meal, a source of focus and stamina during intense study sessions and sports competitions.

This chapter celebrates the power of nourishment and the joy of discovering meals that fuel the body and elevate the spirit. As you and your young chefs prepare this flavorful baked salmon together, may you savor the appreciation for wholesome nourishment and the happiness that comes from enjoying a delicious and nutritious feast. Bon appétit!

Baked Salmon with Lemon and Herbs:

BAKED SALMON WITH LEMON AND HERBS

Ingredients:
- 2 salmon fillets
- 1 lemon
- Fresh herbs (e.g., dill, thyme, or parsley)
- Salt and pepper to taste
- Olive oil for drizzling

Instructions:

1. Preheat your oven to 375°F (190°C) and line a baking sheet with parchment paper.

2. Place the salmon fillets on the prepared baking sheet.

3. Cut the lemon into thin slices.

4. Squeeze some lemon juice over the salmon fillets, and then place a few lemon slices on top of each fillet.

5. Finely chop the fresh herbs, and sprinkle them over the salmon.

6. Season the salmon with a pinch of salt and pepper to taste.

7. Drizzle a little olive oil over the salmon to keep it moist during baking.

8. Bake the salmon in the preheated oven for about 12-15 minutes or until the salmon is cooked through and flakes easily with a fork.

9. Once the salmon is done, remove it from the oven and let it rest for a minute before serving.

10. Serve the baked salmon with lemon and herbs as a flavorful and healthy main course.

**Inspire young chefs to appreciate the natural flavors of ingredients like salmon and to find joy in creating delicious and healthy dishes. Cooking is a journey of discovering the beauty of flavors. Happy baking and savoring the taste of the sea!

16

Whole-Grain Pasta with Marinara Sauce and Veggies

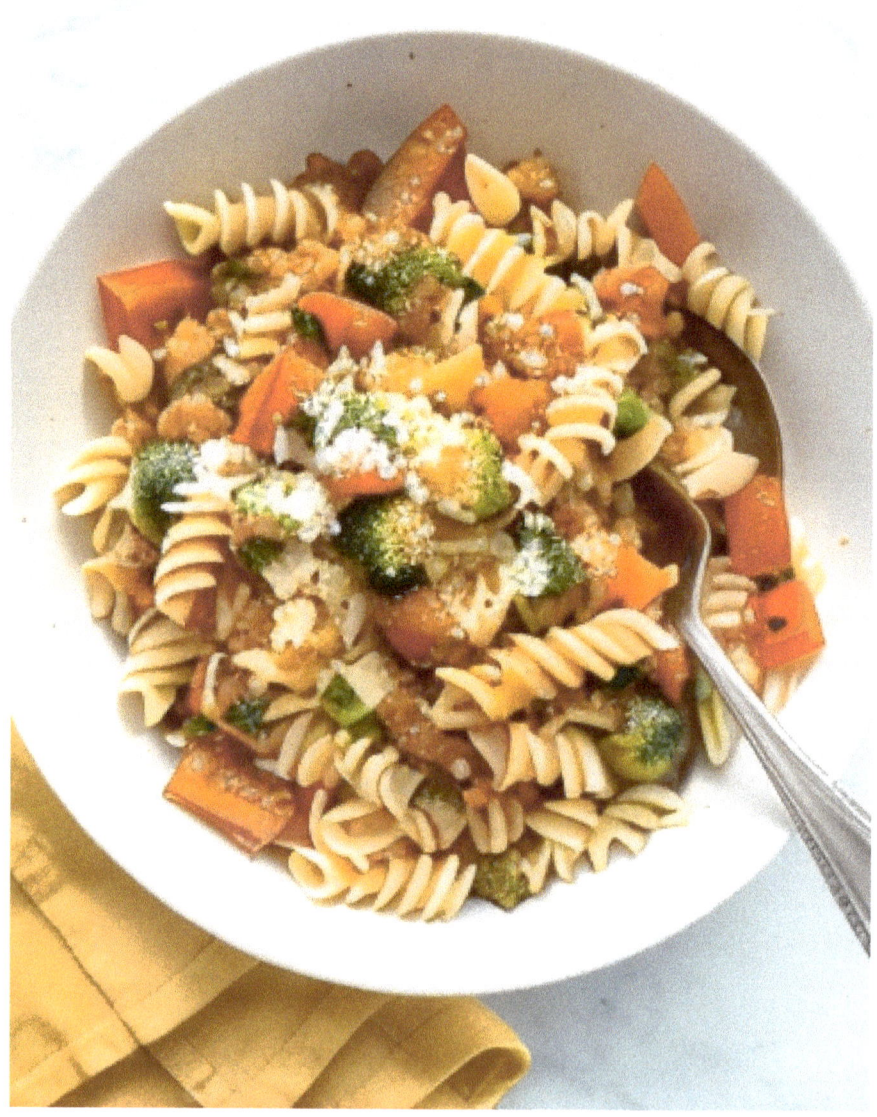

Whole-Grain Pasta with Marinara Sauce and Veggies

"*In every pasta bowl, you hold the power to create a medley of flavors and colors. Embrace the art of combining tastes, and with every bite, feel the pride of your culinary creation!*"

WHOLE-GRAIN PASTA WITH MARINARA SAUCE AND VEGGIES

- *Divine Family Unit*

In our kitchen, there's a heartwarming tale of appreciation and delight that inspired my sons to embrace the wholesome goodness of Whole-Grain Pasta with Marinara Sauce and Veggies. This meal not only makes their taste buds dance with joy but also holds a special place on the cover of this cookbook—a true testament to its delicious and feel-good magic.

As we set out to create a meal that would satisfy both their palates and their bodies, we chose whole-grain pasta, rich in fiber and essential nutrients, as the star of this dish.

With enthusiasm, they tossed the whole-grain pasta into boiling water, eagerly anticipating its al dente perfection. I explained how whole-grain pasta provided a steady release of energy, keeping them fueled and focused throughout the day.

As the pasta was cooked, we prepared a flavorful marinara sauce with ripe tomatoes, aromatic garlic, and fragrant basil. The tomatoes offered a burst of lycopene, a powerful antioxidant that would nourish their bodies and boost their immune systems.

With a medley of colorful vegetables—vibrant bell peppers, tender zucchini, and crisp broccoli—the sauce came to life, creating a delightful and nutritious symphony of flavors.

As they twirled the whole-grain pasta on their forks and spooned the rich marinara sauce with veggies, a sense of satisfaction filled the room. The meal not only tasted divine but also made them feel great after eating it—a perfect harmony of taste and well-being.

From that moment on, Whole-Grain Pasta with Marinara Sauce and Veggies became their go-to meal, a true crowd-pleaser that delighted their taste buds and filled them with nourishing goodness.

This chapter celebrates the magic of wholesome ingredients and the joy of creating meals that make you feel great from the inside out. As you and your young chefs prepare this delightful whole-grain pasta dish together, may you savor the appreciation for wholesome goodness and the happiness that comes from sharing a meal that nourishes both body and soul. Bon appétit!

Whole-Grain Pasta with Marinara Sauce and Veggies:

Ingredients:
 - Whole-grain pasta (spaghetti, penne, or your favorite shape)
 - Marinara sauce (store-bought or homemade)
 - Assorted vegetables (e.g., bell peppers, zucchini, cherry tomatoes, etc.)

Instructions:

1. Cook the whole-grain pasta according to the package instructions. Be sure to ask an adult for help with boiling water and handling the hot pasta.

2. While the pasta is cooking, wash and prepare the assorted vegetables. Cut them into bite-sized pieces or slices.

3. In a separate saucepan, warm the marinara sauce over low heat until it's heated through.

4. Add the prepared vegetables to the warm marinara sauce, and let them simmer for a few minutes until they are tender-crisp.

5. Once the pasta is cooked, drain it in a colander.

6. Return the drained pasta to the pot, and pour the marinara sauce with vegetables over the pasta. Toss everything together until the pasta is coated

WHOLE-GRAIN PASTA WITH MARINARA SAUCE AND VEGGIES

with the sauce.

7. Serve the whole-grain pasta with marinara sauce and veggies as a delicious and nutritious meal.

**Inspire young chefs to appreciate the art of combining flavors and colors in their pasta dishes, and to take pride in their culinary creations. Cooking is an opportunity for creativity and delight in delicious outcomes. Happy cooking and pasta medley creating!

17

Fruit Smoothie with Yogurt and Spinach

FRUIT SMOOTHIE WITH YOGURT AND SPINACH

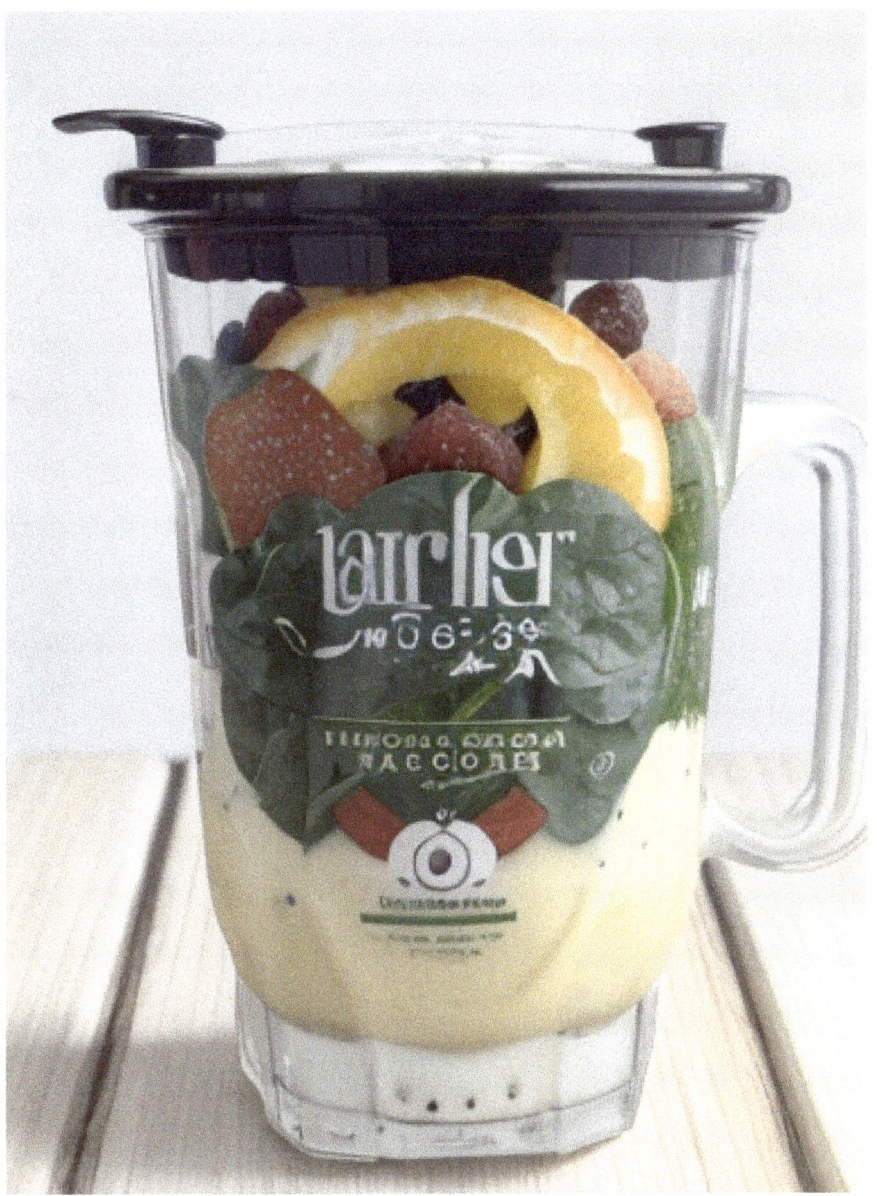

Fruit Smoothie with Yogurt and Spinach

"*In every smoothie, you have the power to blend health and happiness. Embrace the colors of nature, and with every sip, feel the joy of your culinary creation!*" - *Coach Rae*

In our culinary journey, there's a tale of deliciousness and well-being that led my sons to embrace the vibrant goodness of a Fruit Smoothie with Yogurt and Spinach. This quick and delightful meal not only satisfies their taste buds but also leaves them feeling great and energized.

As we set out to create a refreshing and nutritious smoothie, we gathered an array of colorful fruits—sweet bananas, succulent strawberries, and juicy blueberries, each chosen for their natural sweetness and abundance of vitamins.

To boost the nutritional content, we added a handful of vibrant spinach leaves, a powerhouse of essential nutrients that would nourish their growing bodies.

With excitement, they blended the fruits and spinach with creamy yogurt, creating a velvety and flavorful concoction that was both indulgent and wholesome.

I explained how the fruits provided a burst of vitamins and antioxidants, while the yogurt offered a creamy and probiotic-rich base that would support their digestive health.

As they sipped on the Fruit Smoothie with Yogurt and Spinach, their eyes lit up with delight. The delightful blend of flavors left them feeling refreshed and energized—a perfect pick-me-up for any time of the day.

From that moment on, the Fruit Smoothie with Yogurt and Spinach became their go-to quick meal, a delicious and nutritious treat that brightened their day and nourished their bodies.

This chapter celebrates the joy of vibrant flavors and the magic of creating nutritious meals that make you feel great inside and out. As you and your young chefs prepare this delightful fruit smoothie together, may you savor the deliciousness and the happiness that comes from enjoying a refreshing and nourishing beverage. Bon appétit!

Fruit Smoothie with Yogurt and Spinach:

Ingredients:
- Assorted fruits (e.g., bananas, berries, mango, etc.)
- 1 cup plain or flavored yogurt
- Handful of fresh spinach leaves
- 1/2 cup milk (or dairy-free alternative)
- Honey or maple syrup for sweetness (optional)

Instructions:

1. Wash and prepare the assorted fruits. Peel and slice them into small pieces.

2. In a blender, combine the sliced fruits, plain or flavored yogurt, fresh spinach leaves, and milk.

3. Blend everything until you have a smooth and creamy consistency. If you prefer a thicker smoothie, you can add more frozen fruits or ice cubes.

4. Taste the smoothie and add a drizzle of honey or maple syrup for sweetness, if desired.

5. Blend again briefly to mix in the sweetener.

6. Pour the fruit smoothie into glasses or bottles for serving.

7. If you like, you can garnish the smoothie with a small piece of fruit or a fresh spinach leaf.

8. Your fruit smoothie with yogurt and spinach is ready to enjoy!

**Inspire young chefs to see their smoothie as a colorful and nutritious blend of nature's goodness, and to take joy in creating healthy and delicious drinks. Cooking is a celebration of health and happiness. Happy blending and sipping the joy!

18

Stuffed Bell Peppers with Lean Ground Turkey

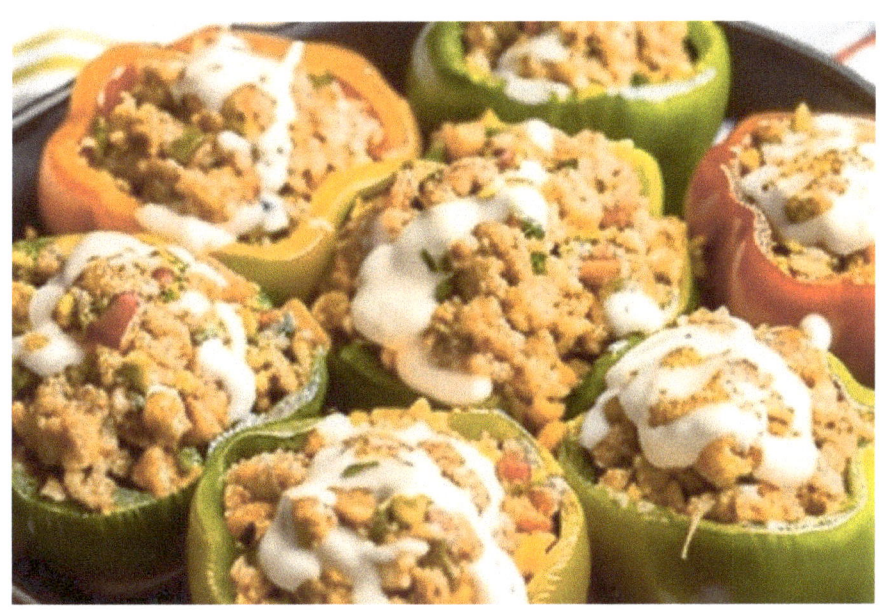

Stuffed Bell Peppers with Lean Ground Turkey

"I*n every stuffed bell pepper, you have the power to create a balanced delight and a culinary masterpiece. Embrace the art of stuffing, and* *with every bite, feel the excitement of your culinary creation!" - Uncle T*

In our kitchen, there's a heartwarming tale of discovery and cherished memories that led my sons to fall in love with the delightful taste of Stuffed Bell Peppers with Lean Ground Turkey. This quick and delicious meal not only satisfies their appetites but also brings back fond moments spent with loved ones.

It all began during a visit to their uncle's house, where they were introduced to the magic of stuffed bell peppers. The aroma of sizzling lean ground turkey and fragrant herbs filled the air, tantalizing their taste buds with anticipation.

As they watched their uncle prepare the meal, he shared the magic of combining lean ground turkey with a medley of colorful bell peppers. The peppers, chosen for their sweet and vibrant flavors, were the perfect vessel to hold the savory goodness of the turkey filling.

With excitement, they helped their uncle stuff the bell peppers with the seasoned lean ground turkey mixture, eager to taste the delicious creation they had crafted together.

As the stuffed bell peppers baked in the oven, the flavors melded together, creating a comforting and wholesome dish that was both nutritious and scrumptious.

When they took their first bites, their taste buds were met with a delightful combination of tender turkey and sweet bell peppers. The meal reminded them of the time spent with loved ones, cherishing the joy of being together and enjoying each other's company.

From that moment on, Stuffed Bell Peppers with Lean Ground Turkey became a cherished recipe, a meal that not only satisfied their hunger but also brought back warm and cherished memories.

This chapter celebrates the joy of discovering new flavors and the magic of creating meals that evoke cherished moments with loved ones. As you and your young chefs prepare these delightful stuffed bell peppers together, may you savor the joy of creating cherished memories and the happiness that comes from sharing a delicious and heartwarming meal with family and friends. Bon appétit!

Stuffed Bell Peppers with Lean Ground Chicken:

Ingredients:
- 4 bell peppers (assorted colors)
- 1 pound lean ground chicken
- 1 cup cooked quinoa or brown rice
- 1/2 cup diced tomatoes (canned or fresh)
- 1/2 cup diced onion
- 1/2 cup diced zucchini
- 1/2 cup diced mushrooms
- 1 clove garlic, minced
- 1 teaspoon olive oil
- 1 teaspoon dried herbs (e.g., basil, oregano, or thyme)
- Salt and pepper to taste
- Grated cheese for topping (optional)

Instructions:

1. Preheat your oven to 375°F (190°C).

2. Cut the tops off the bell peppers and remove the seeds and membranes.

3. Wash the bell peppers inside and out, and place them in a baking dish.

4. In a skillet over medium heat, add olive oil and sauté the diced onions until they become translucent.

5. Add the minced garlic and cook for another minute.

6. Stir in the diced zucchini and mushrooms, and cook until they soften slightly.

7. Add the lean ground chicken to the skillet, breaking it up with a spatula as it cooks.

8. Season the mixture with dried herbs, salt, and pepper.

9. Once the chicken is cooked through, add the cooked quinoa or brown rice and diced tomatoes. Mix everything until well combined.

10. Stuff each bell pepper with the chicken and quinoa mixture.

11. If you like, sprinkle some grated cheese on top of each stuffed pepper.

12. Cover the baking dish with foil, and bake the stuffed bell peppers in the preheated oven for about 20-25 minutes, or until the peppers are tender.

13. Remove the foil, and bake for an additional 5 minutes to melt the cheese (if using) and add a touch of crispiness.

14. Let the stuffed bell peppers cool for a moment before serving.

**Inspire young chefs to appreciate the art of stuffing and balancing flavors in their stuffed bell peppers, and to take pride in their culinary creations. Cooking is an opportunity for creativity and creating delightful dishes. Happy stuffing and culinary mastery!

19

Veggie and Cheese Quesadillas

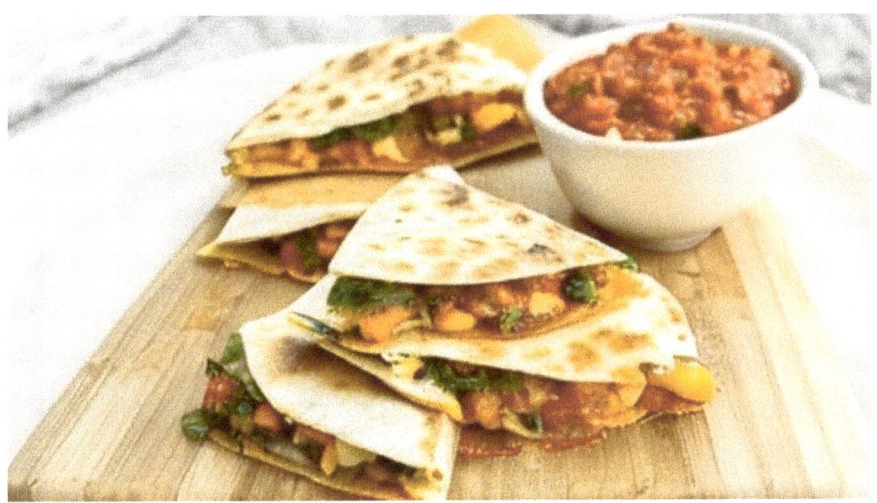

Veggie and Cheese Quesadillas

"*In every quesadilla, you hold the power to create a taste of Mexico and a culinary fiesta. Embrace the art of melting flavors, and with every bite, feel the vibe of your culinary creation!*" - Papa True Ju

In our culinary journey, there's a tale of immediate love and sunny memories that led my sons to embrace the mouthwatering delight of Veggie and Cheese

Quesadillas. This quick and delicious meal not only captivated their taste buds but also transported them to bright and sunny California days in the Bay Area.

Growing up in the Bay Area, they discovered the magic of quesadillas while soaking up the warm California sun. The vibrant colors of the vegetables and the melting cheese inside the crispy tortilla were a feast for their eyes.

As they savored their first bites, the flavors exploded on their taste buds—tender sautéed vegetables combined with gooey melted cheese, creating a harmonious and delectable filling.

The ingredients were carefully selected to ensure a delicious and nutritious blend. Colorful bell peppers and zucchini provided a medley of vitamins and minerals, while the cheese added a creamy and indulgent touch to the dish.

As they enjoyed the Veggie and Cheese Quesadillas under the sunny skies of California, the meal became synonymous with the joy of exploring new places and cherishing the moments spent with loved ones.

From that moment on, Veggie and Cheese Quesadillas became a favorite meal, a reminder of bright and sunny California days and the warmth of family and friends.

This chapter celebrates the joy of culinary discoveries and the magic of creating meals that evoke cherished memories. As you and your young chefs prepare these delightful quesadillas together, may you savor the immediate love and happiness that comes from sharing a delicious and sunny-inspired meal. Bon appétit!

Veggie and Cheese Quesadillas:

VEGGIE AND CHEESE QUESADILLAS

Ingredients:
- Whole wheat or corn tortillas
- Shredded cheese (e.g., cheddar, mozzarella, or a blend)
- Assorted vegetables (e.g., bell peppers, onions, spinach, etc.)
- Olive oil or butter for cooking

Instructions:

1. Wash and prepare the assorted vegetables. Cut them into thin slices or small pieces.

2. In a non-stick skillet over medium heat, add a drizzle of olive oil or a small amount of butter.

3. Place one tortilla in the skillet, and sprinkle a generous amount of shredded cheese on half of the tortilla.

4. Add a layer of assorted vegetables on top of the cheese.

5. Fold the tortilla in half, covering the cheese and vegetables, to create a half-moon shape.

6. Press the quesadilla down gently with a spatula to help the cheese melt and seal the filling.

7. Cook the quesadilla for 2-3 minutes on each side, or until the tortilla becomes golden brown and crispy, and the cheese is melted.

8. Remove the cooked quesadilla from the skillet, and let it cool for a moment before slicing.

9. Repeat the process for additional quesadillas.

10. Slice the quesadillas into wedges and serve them as a delicious and satisfying meal.

**Inspire young chefs to appreciate the art of melting flavors and creating a culinary fiesta in their veggie and cheese quesadillas, and to take joy in their culinary creations. Cooking is an opportunity for creativity and a delicious adventure. Happy quesadilla-making and culinary fiesta!

20

Mediterranean Chickpea Salad

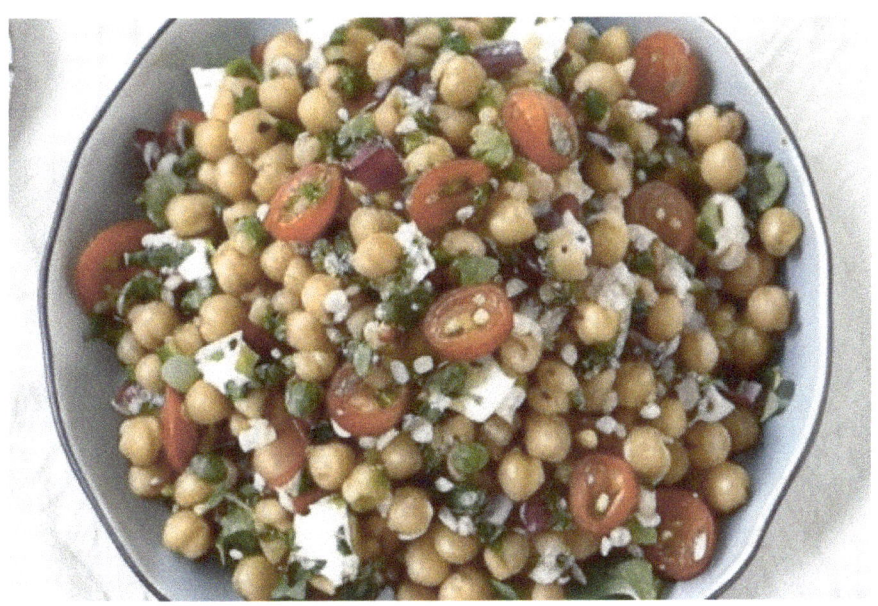

Mediterranean Chickpea Salad

"In every chickpea salad, you have the power to blend flavors from the Mediterranean and create a taste of sunshine. Embrace the magic of wholesome ingredients, and with every bite, feel the pride of your culinary creation!" - Divine Family Unit

In our kitchen, there's a tale of hesitant exploration and newfound appreciation that led my sons to embrace the delightful flavors of Mediterranean Chickpea Salad. This quick and delicious meal, once met with uncertainty, has now become one that they joyfully prepare and savor.

At first, they were unsure about trying the Mediterranean Chickpea Salad, as the flavors of the Mediterranean seemed foreign to their taste buds. However, I encouraged them to take a leap of faith and explore the magic of this vibrant salad.

As they combined the tender chickpeas with colorful cherry tomatoes, crisp cucumbers, and tangy feta cheese, a delightful medley of flavors emerged. The chickpeas provided a hearty and protein-rich base, while the cherry tomatoes and cucumbers added a burst of freshness and vitamins.

With a drizzle of zesty lemon juice and a sprinkle of aromatic herbs like oregano and parsley, the salad came to life, offering a symphony of Mediterranean flavors that danced on their taste buds.

As they took their first bites, they were pleasantly surprised by the harmonious blend of flavors and textures. The once hesitant exploration had turned into an appreciation for the delightful taste and nourishment that the Mediterranean Chickpea Salad provided.

From that moment on, Mediterranean Chickpea Salad became a beloved dish, one that they now joyfully prepare and savor. The salad not only delights their palates but also offers a taste of the Mediterranean that they cherish.

This chapter celebrates the joy of trying new flavors and the magic of creating meals that open doors to culinary delights. As you and your young chefs prepare this delightful Mediterranean Chickpea Salad together, may you savor the joy of newfound appreciation and the happiness that comes from embracing culinary adventures. Bon appétit!

Mediterranean Chickpea Salad:

Ingredients:
- 1 can chickpeas (15 ounces), drained and rinsed
- 1 cup cherry tomatoes, halved
- 1 cucumber, diced
- 1/4 cup diced red onion
- 1/4 cup chopped Kalamata olives
- 1/4 cup crumbled feta cheese
- 2 tablespoons extra-virgin olive oil
- 1 tablespoon lemon juice
- 1 teaspoon dried oregano
- Salt and pepper to taste
- Fresh parsley or basil for garnish (optional)

Instructions:

1. In a large mixing bowl, combine the chickpeas, halved cherry tomatoes, diced cucumber, diced red onion, chopped Kalamata olives, and crumbled feta cheese.

2. In a separate small bowl, whisk together the extra-virgin olive oil, lemon juice, dried oregano, salt, and pepper to create the dressing.

3. Pour the dressing over the chickpea mixture and gently toss until everything is well coated.

4. Taste the salad and adjust the seasoning if needed.

5. If you like, garnish the Mediterranean chickpea salad with fresh parsley or basil for added freshness and presentation.

6. Serve the salad immediately or refrigerate it for later enjoyment.

**Inspire young chefs to appreciate the magic of blending flavors from the Mediterranean in their chickpea salad, and to take pride in creating a dish that brings a taste of sunshine to their meal. Cooking is a delightful journey of flavors and sunshine. Happy salad-making and culinary creativity!

21

Turkey and Vegetable Kebabs

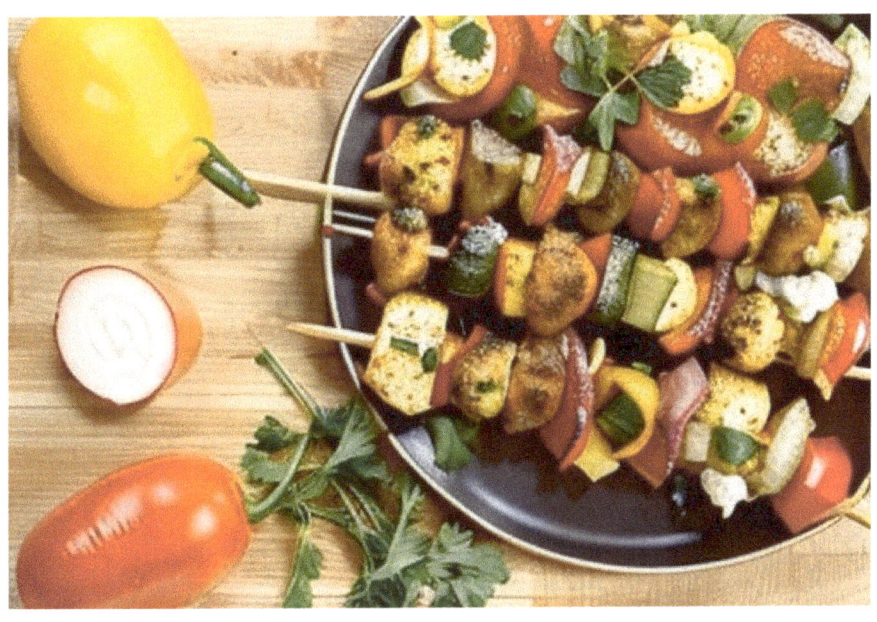

Turkey and Vegetable Kebabs

"In every kebab, you hold the power to thread joy and health onto a skewer. Embrace the harmony of tastes, and with every bite, feel the pride of your culinary creation!" - Coach Rae

In our kitchen, there's a tale of unwavering enthusiasm and culinary delight that led my sons to embrace the joy of preparing and savoring Turkey and Vegetable Kebabs. This delectable and fun meal has become a beloved favorite, one they don't miss a chance to enjoy.

The magic begins as they gather tender turkey chunks, chosen for their lean and protein-packed goodness, and an assortment of vibrant vegetables—colorful bell peppers, juicy cherry tomatoes, and tender zucchini, each providing a burst of flavors and essential nutrients.

As they thread the turkey and vegetables onto skewers, they delight in the art of creating colorful and appetizing kebabs. The skewers become a canvas for their culinary creativity, joyous exploration of taste, and presentation.

With a sprinkle of aromatic herbs and a drizzle of olive oil, the kebabs come to life, promising a delightful and nourishing feast.

As they grill the kebabs to perfection, the enticing aroma fills the air, inviting everyone to gather around for a shared moment of culinary delight.

When they take their first bites, their faces light up with joy. The tender turkey mingles with the vibrant vegetables, creating a harmonious dance of flavors and textures that they savor with every mouthful.

From that moment on, Turkey and Vegetable Kebabs became a favorite meal, one they joyfully prepare and savor whenever the opportunity arises.

This chapter celebrates the joy of culinary creativity and the magic of creating meals that bring smiles to everyone's faces. As you and your young chefs prepare these delightful kebabs together, may you savor the unwavering enthusiasm and happiness that comes from enjoying a delicious and fun-filled meal. Bon appétit!

Turkey and Vegetable Kebabs:

Ingredients:
- 1 pound ground turkey
- Assorted vegetables (e.g., bell peppers, cherry tomatoes, zucchini, etc.)
- Wooden or metal skewers
- Olive oil
- Salt and pepper to taste
- Optional seasonings (e.g., garlic powder, paprika, or cumin)

Instructions:

1. If you're using wooden skewers, soak them in water for about 30 minutes to prevent them from burning during cooking.

2. In a large mixing bowl, season the ground turkey with salt, pepper, and any optional seasonings of your choice. Mix everything together until well combined.

3. Wash and prepare the assorted vegetables. Cut them into bite-sized pieces.

4. Take a small amount of seasoned ground turkey and shape it into a small ball.

5. Slide the turkey ball onto a skewer, followed by a piece of vegetable. Repeat the process, alternating between turkey and vegetables until the skewer is filled.

6. Repeat the skewering process with the remaining ground turkey and vegetables.

7. Preheat a grill or stovetop grill pan over medium heat.

8. Drizzle a little olive oil over the turkey and vegetable kebabs to prevent sticking and add extra flavor.

9. Grill the kebabs for about 10-12 minutes, turning them occasionally to ensure even cooking, until the turkey is fully cooked and no longer pink.

10. Once the kebabs are cooked, remove them from the grill and let them cool for a moment before serving.

11. Serve the turkey and vegetable kebabs as a delicious and protein-rich meal.

**Inspire young chefs to see their kebabs as a harmony of flavors and a delightful combination of joy and health, and to take pride in creating a protein-rich and delicious meal. Cooking is a chance to thread happiness and health into every dish. Happy skewering and culinary delight!

22

Broccoli and Cheese Stuffed Potatoes

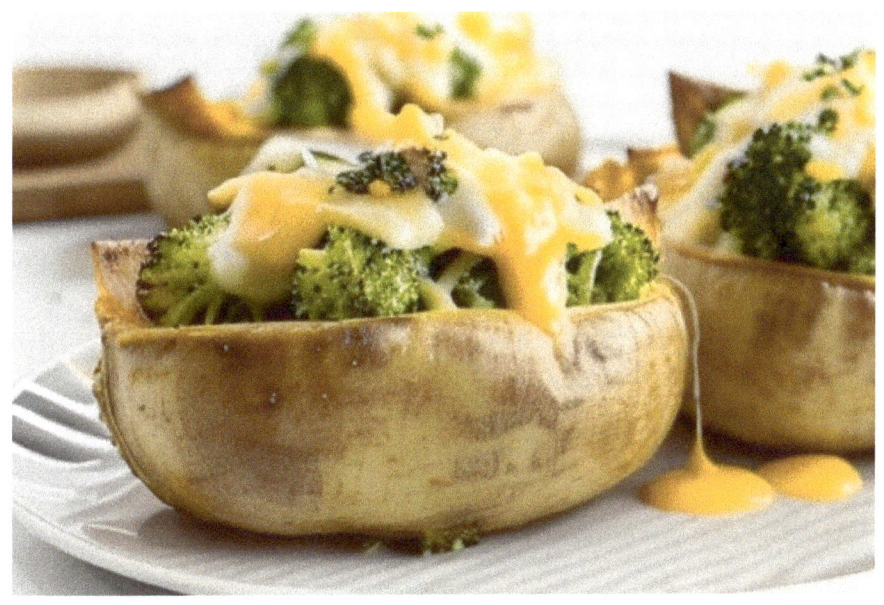

Broccoli and Cheese Stuffed Potatoes

"In every stuffed potato, you hold the power to create a comfort-filled crater and a culinary hug. Embrace the warmth of your meal, and with every bite, feel inspired by your culinary creation!" - Papa True

Ju

In our culinary journey, there's a heartwarming tale of shared moments and delightful simplicity that led my sons to embrace the delicious taste of Broccoli and Cheese Stuffed Potatoes. This comforting and flavorful meal holds a special place in their hearts, inspired by a cherished evening watching their Papa prepare it.

One evening, they watched with curiosity as I carefully baked tender potatoes until they were fluffy and inviting. The potatoes, chosen for their versatility and earthy flavor, were the perfect canvas for the delightful stuffing.

With excitement, they helped me prepare a luscious stuffing of tender broccoli florets and a generous amount of gooey cheese. The combination of nutritious broccoli and savory cheese created a medley of flavors that they couldn't resist.

As they eagerly spooned the stuffing into the baked potatoes, the kitchen filled with a delightful aroma that set the stage for a satisfying feast.

When they took their first bites, their faces lit up with delight. The tender potato mingled with the flavorful stuffing, creating a symphony of taste that they savored with each mouthful.

From that moment on, Broccoli and Cheese Stuffed Potatoes became a cherished meal, a comforting and flavorful treat that they have fallen in love with.

This chapter celebrates the joy of shared moments in the kitchen and the magic of creating meals that warm the heart and soul. As you and your young chefs prepare these delightful stuffed potatoes together, may you savor the simplicity and deliciousness that comes from enjoying a comforting and nourishing meal with loved ones. Bon appétit!

Broccoli and Cheese Stuffed Potatoes:

BROCCOLI AND CHEESE STUFFED POTATOES

Ingredients:
- 4 large baking potatoes
- 1 cup steamed broccoli florets
- 1 cup shredded cheddar cheese (or any favorite cheese)
- 1/2 cup sour cream (or Greek yogurt for a lighter option)
- Salt and pepper to taste
- Olive oil or melted butter for brushing

Instructions:

1. Preheat your oven to 400°F (200°C).

2. Wash the potatoes thoroughly and pat them dry with a paper towel.

3. Using a fork, pierce the potatoes a few times to create small holes. This will allow steam to escape while baking.

4. Rub the potatoes with a little olive oil or melted butter to create a crispy skin during baking.

5. Place the potatoes directly on the oven rack or on a baking sheet, and bake them in the preheated oven for about 45-60 minutes or until they are tender when pierced with a fork.

6. While the potatoes are baking, steam the broccoli florets until they are tender-crisp.

7. Once the potatoes are done, let them cool slightly for handling.

8. Carefully slice off the top of each potato and scoop out the flesh, leaving a potato shell.

9. In a mixing bowl, mash the potato flesh with a fork.

10. Add the steamed broccoli, shredded cheddar cheese, and sour cream to the mashed potatoes. Mix everything together until well combined.

11. Season the potato mixture with salt and pepper to taste.

12. Stuff each potato shell with the broccoli and cheese mixture.

13. Place the stuffed potatoes back in the oven for an additional 5-10 minutes, or until the cheese is melted and bubbly.

14. Remove the stuffed potatoes from the oven, and let them cool slightly before serving.

**Inspire young chefs to appreciate the warmth and comfort they bring to their stuffed potatoes, and to take pride in their culinary creations. Cooking is an opportunity to create delicious comfort and culinary hugs. Happy stuffing and enjoying the culinary warmth!

23

Hummus and Veggie Platter

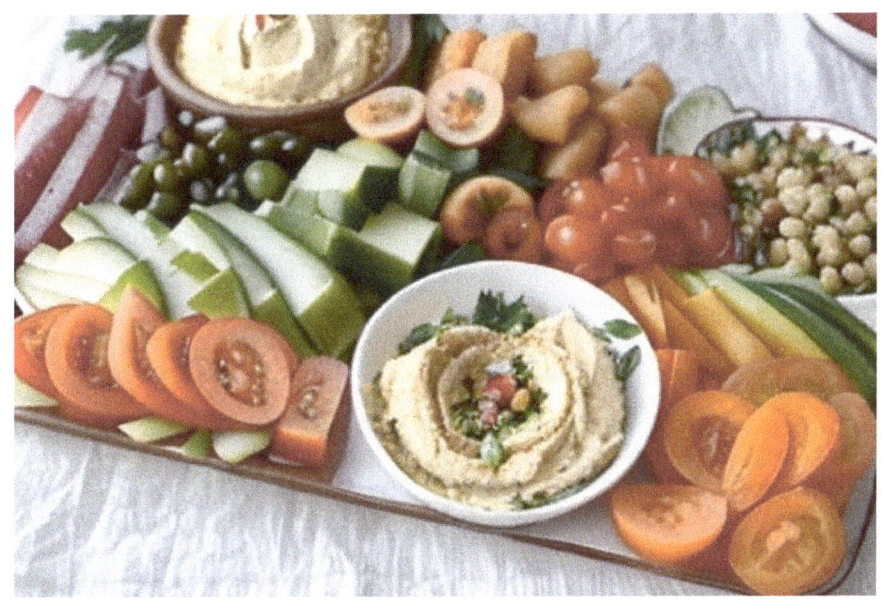

Hummus and Veggie Platter

"*In every hummus dip and veggie crunch, you have the power to create a colorful masterpiece and a culinary celebration. Embrace the joy of sharing and the pride of your culinary creation!*" - *Divine Family Unit*

In our kitchen, there's a tale of fascination and culinary discovery that led my sons to embrace the delightful taste of a Hummus and Veggie Platter. This vibrant and wholesome meal holds a special place in their hearts, inspired by a captivating afternoon watching their Papa prepare it.

One sunny afternoon, they gathered around as I crafted a creamy and flavorful hummus, blending chickpeas with tahini, lemon juice, and a touch of garlic. The hummus, chosen for its rich and nutty taste, became the star of the platter.

With enthusiasm, they helped me prepare an array of colorful vegetables—crisp carrot sticks, crunchy cucumber slices, and sweet bell pepper strips. The vegetables offered a medley of colors and vitamins, providing a delightful and nutritious pairing with the hummus.

As they artfully arranged the veggies around the creamy hummus, the platter came to life, promising a delightful and satisfying snack that would tantalize their taste buds.

When they took their first dips, their eyes widened with delight. The creamy hummus mingled with the fresh and crunchy vegetables, creating a symphony of flavors and textures that they couldn't get enough of.

From that moment on, Hummus and Veggie Platter became a cherished meal, a fascinating and wholesome treat that they have fallen in love with.

This chapter celebrates the joy of culinary discovery and the magic of creating meals that spark fascination and delight. As you and your young chefs prepare this delightful hummus and veggie platter together, may you savor the vibrant flavors and the happiness that comes from enjoying a delicious and nourishing meal. Bon appétit!

Hummus and Veggie Platter:

HUMMUS AND VEGGIE PLATTER

Ingredients:
- Store-bought or homemade hummus
- Assorted vegetables (e.g., carrots, cucumber, bell peppers, cherry tomatoes, etc.)
- Pita bread or whole-grain crackers for serving

Instructions:

1. Wash and prepare the assorted vegetables. Cut them into thin sticks or bite-sized pieces, suitable for dipping.

2. If you're using store-bought hummus, transfer it to a serving bowl. If you prefer homemade hummus, prepare it ahead of time and place it in a bowl.

3. Arrange the prepared vegetables around the hummus bowl on a platter or a large serving plate.

4. If you have pita bread or whole-grain crackers, you can place them on the platter as well for dipping.

5. Your Hummus and Veggie Platter is now ready to serve!

**Inspire young chefs to appreciate the joy of sharing their Hummus and Veggie Platter, and to take pride in creating a colorful and nutritious culinary masterpiece. Cooking is an opportunity to celebrate and share delightful flavors. Happy dipping and culinary celebration!

24

Mini Turkey Meatloaf with Mashed Cauliflower

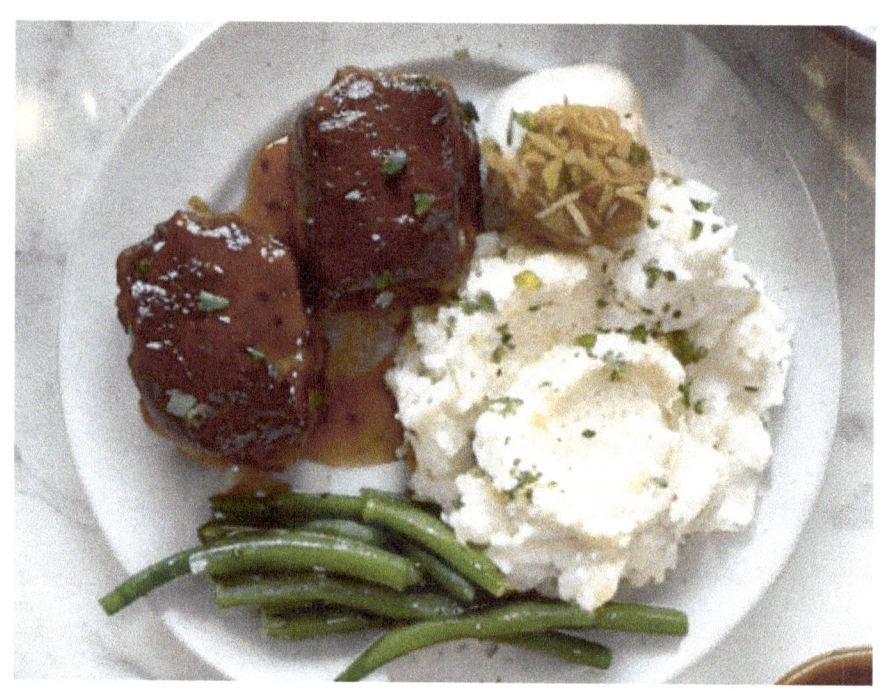

Mini Turkey Meatloaf with Mashed Cauliflower

MINI TURKEY MEATLOAF WITH MASHED CAULIFLOWER

"*In every mini meatloaf and mashed cauliflower, you hold the power to create a comforting feast and a culinary triumph. Embrace the art of nourishing flavors, and with every bite, feel the awesomeness of your culinary creation!*" - Coach Rae

In our culinary journey, there's a tale of determination and savory success that led my sons to embrace the fascinating taste of Mini Turkey Meatloaf with Mashed Cauliflower. This comforting and flavorful meal holds a special place in their hearts, inspired by their perseverance and the joy of mastering a delicious dish.

With an eagerness to take on a new cooking challenge, my sons set out to create a mini turkey meatloaf that would be both wholesome and delectable. They carefully selected lean ground turkey, chosen for its rich protein content and tender texture.

As they mixed the turkey with aromatic herbs, a medley of flavors emerged, promising a savory and satisfying meatloaf that would delight their taste buds.

With patience and practice, they molded the turkey mixture into mini loaves, carefully ensuring that each loaf was perfectly shaped and seasoned to perfection.

Meanwhile, they prepared mashed cauliflower—a clever and nutritious twist to traditional mashed potatoes. The cauliflower, chosen for its tender texture and mild taste, became a creamy and wholesome companion to the meatloaf.

As they proudly presented their mini turkey meatloaves with a dollop of mashed cauliflower on the side, their faces beamed with joy. The meatloaf, tender and flavorful, paired harmoniously with the creamy mashed cauliflower.

When they took their first bites, they knew all their hard work had paid off. The mini turkey meatloaf, infused with aromatic herbs and spices, mingled with the velvety mashed cauliflower, creating a symphony of taste that they savored with every mouthful.

From that moment on, Mini Turkey Meatloaf with Mashed Cauliflower became a cherished meal, a fascinating and wholesome treat that they have fallen in love with.

This chapter celebrates the joy of perseverance and the magic of creating meals that bring a sense of accomplishment and happiness. As you and your young chefs prepare these delightful mini turkey meatloaves with mashed cauliflower together, may you savor the determination and the deliciousness that comes from mastering a savory and wholesome meal. Bon appétit!

Mini Turkey Meatloaf with Mashed Cauliflower:

Ingredients for Mini Turkey Meatloaf:
- 1 pound ground turkey
- 1/2 cup breadcrumbs
- 1/4 cup finely chopped onion
- 1/4 cup finely chopped bell pepper
- 1/4 cup ketchup or barbecue sauce
- 1 large egg, lightly beaten
- 1 teaspoon Worcestershire sauce
- 1/2 teaspoon garlic powder
- Salt and pepper to taste

Ingredients for Mashed Cauliflower:
- 1 medium head of cauliflower, cut into florets
- 2 tablespoons butter or olive oil
- 1/4 cup milk (or dairy-free alternative)
- Salt and pepper to taste

MINI TURKEY MEATLOAF WITH MASHED CAULIFLOWER

Instructions for Mini Turkey Meatloaf:

1. Preheat your oven to 375°F (190°C).

2. In a large mixing bowl, combine ground turkey, breadcrumbs, finely chopped onion, bell pepper, ketchup or barbecue sauce, lightly beaten egg, Worcestershire sauce, garlic powder, salt, and pepper.

3. Mix everything until all the ingredients are well incorporated.

4. Divide the turkey mixture into equal portions and shape them into mini meatloaves.

5. Place the mini meatloaves on a baking sheet lined with parchment paper.

6. Bake the mini meatloaves in the preheated oven for about 25-30 minutes or until they are cooked through and reach an internal temperature of 165°F (74°C).

Instructions for Mashed Cauliflower:

1. In a large pot, bring water to a boil and add the cauliflower florets.

2. Boil the cauliflower until it is tender, about 10-15 minutes.

3. Drain the cooked cauliflower and return it to the pot.

4. Mash the cauliflower using a potato masher or fork until it reaches your desired consistency.

5. Add butter or olive oil, milk, salt, and pepper to the mashed cauliflower, and continue mashing and mixing until well combined.

6. Taste the mashed cauliflower and adjust the seasoning if needed.

7. Your Mini Turkey Meatloaf with Mashed Cauliflower is now ready to serve!

**Inspire young chefs to appreciate the art of nourishing flavors in their Mini Turkey Meatloaf with Mashed Cauliflower, and to take pride in their culinary triumph. Cooking is an opportunity to create comforting and delicious feasts. Happy cooking and culinary creativity!

25

Brown Rice with Black Beans and Salsa

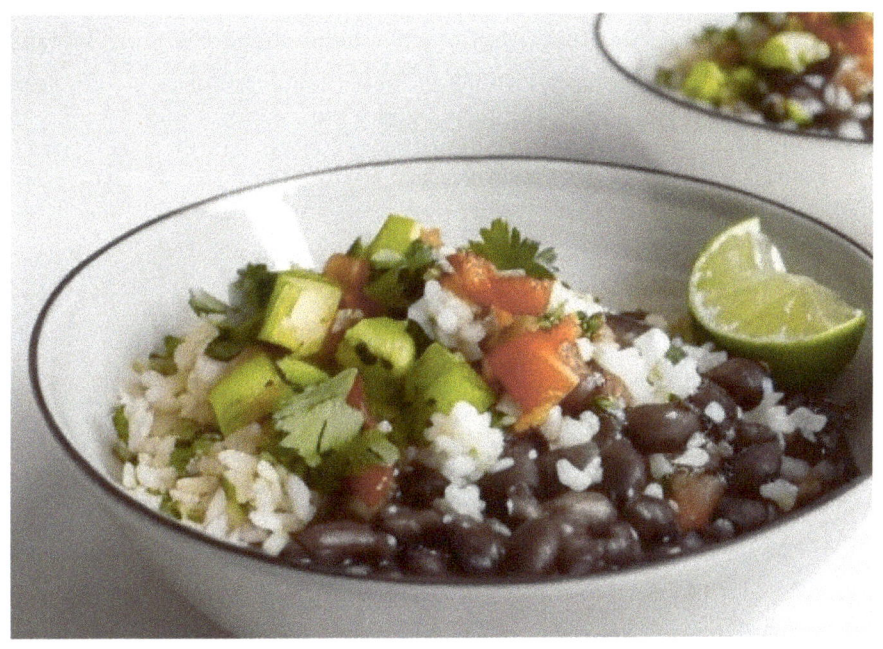

Brown Rice with Black Beans and Salsa

"*In every brown rice bowl, you have the power to blend colors and textures and create a fiesta of flavors. Embrace the joy of culinary harmony, and with each bite, feel the excitement of your culinary creation!" - Divine Family Unit*

In our kitchen, there's a heartwarming tale of learning and cherished family traditions that led my sons to embrace the wonderful taste of Brown Rice with Black Beans and Salsa. This wholesome and flavorful meal holds a special place in their hearts, inspired by the countless times they watched their mother prepare it for the family.

As they gathered around, they observed their mother cook nutty brown rice, chosen for its wholesome goodness and rich fiber content. The rice became the nourishing foundation of the dish.

With curiosity and excitement, they watched as she added tender black beans, rich in protein and essential nutrients. The beans provided a delightful earthy flavor and hearty texture to the dish.

Next came the salsa—a vibrant medley of tomatoes, onions, and cilantro, offering a burst of fresh and tangy flavors. The salsa added a zesty kick, complementing the rice and beans with a delightful balance.

As they eagerly served themselves heaping spoonfuls of Brown Rice with Black Beans and Salsa, they knew they were about to enjoy a wholesome and satisfying meal that had become a beloved family tradition.

When they took their first bites, they smiled with delight. The nutty brown rice mingled with the tender black beans and zesty salsa, creating a symphony of flavors that they savored with each mouthful.

From that moment on, Brown Rice with Black Beans and Salsa became a cherished meal, one that held not only the wonderful taste but also the fond memories of cherished family moments.

This chapter celebrates the joy of learning from loved ones and the magic of creating meals that become beloved family traditions. As you and your young chefs prepare this wholesome and flavorful dish together, may you savor the warmth of family bonds and the deliciousness that comes from enjoying a cherished and nourishing meal. Bon appétit!

Brown Rice with Black Beans and Salsa:

Ingredients:
- 1 cup cooked brown rice
- 1 can black beans (15 ounces), drained and rinsed
- 1 cup salsa (mild, medium, or hot, according to preference)
- Optional toppings: diced avocado, chopped cilantro, shredded cheese, or sour cream

Instructions:

1. If you haven't cooked the brown rice yet, follow the package instructions to cook it until it's tender.

2. In a saucepan, warm the black beans over low heat until they are heated through.

3. In a separate saucepan or microwave, warm the salsa until it's at the desired temperature.

4. In a serving bowl, layer the cooked brown rice, warmed black beans, and salsa.

5. If you like, add any optional toppings, such as diced avocado, chopped cilantro, shredded cheese, or a dollop of sour cream.

6. Mix everything gently until the brown rice, black beans, and salsa are well combined.

7. Your Brown Rice with Black Beans and Salsa is now ready to enjoy!

****Inspire young chefs to appreciate the joy of culinary harmony in their Brown Rice with Black Beans and Salsa, and to take pride in creating a fiesta of flavors with colors and textures. Cooking is an opportunity to create delightful culinary masterpieces. Happy blending and fiesta of flavors!

26

Zucchini Noodles with Tomato Sauce

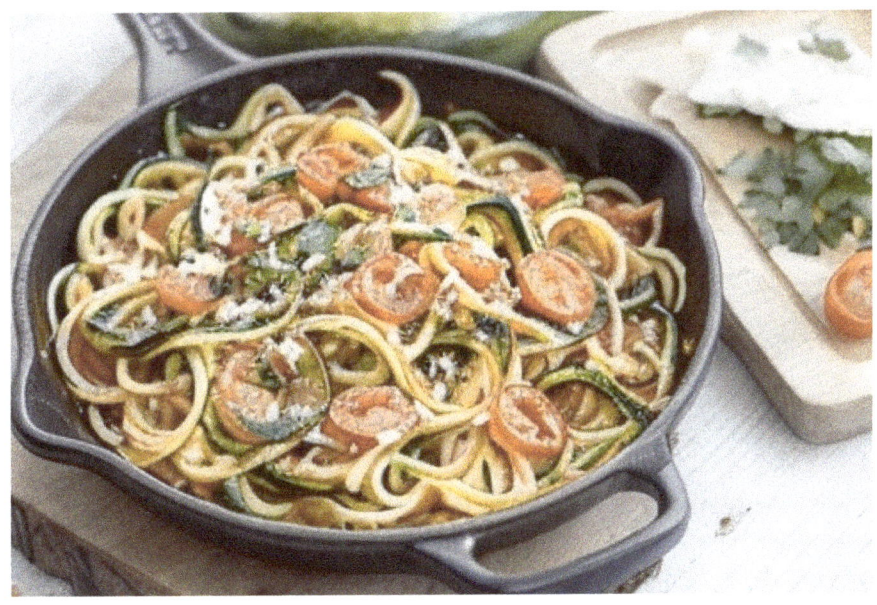

Zucchini Noodles with Tomato Sauce

"*In every zucchini noodle swirl, you hold the power to create a garden of flavors and a culinary canvas. Embrace the art of healthy choices, and with every bite, feel great about your culinary creation!*" - Coach Rae

In our kitchen, there's a tale of appreciation and culinary growth that led my sons to truly savor the well-cooked Zucchini Noodles with Tomato Sauce. This delightful and wholesome meal holds a special place in their hearts, inspired by their mother's masterful preparation and the journey of building their confidence in the kitchen.

At first, Zucchini Noodles with Tomato Sauce posed a challenge, as the delicate zucchini noodles required careful cooking to avoid becoming soggy. The secret lay in achieving the perfect balance, where the zucchini remained tender and firm.

With determination and enthusiasm, they watched their mother prepare this wonderful meal countless times, mastering the art of cooking zucchini noodles to perfection.

She selected fresh zucchini, chosen for its mild flavor and ability to transform into delicate noodles. The zucchini became the star of the dish, offering a wholesome alternative to traditional pasta.

As they observed her combine ripe tomatoes, aromatic herbs, and a hint of garlic into a luscious tomato sauce, they knew they were in for a flavorful and nourishing treat.

With their newfound culinary knowledge, they embarked on creating Zucchini Noodles with Tomato Sauce themselves, their confidence growing exponentially with each attempt.

They carefully cooked the zucchini noodles, ensuring they retained their delightful texture and flavor. The tomato sauce, rich and flavorful, mingled perfectly with the zucchini noodles, creating a symphony of taste that they savored with each mouthful.

From that moment on, Zucchini Noodles with Tomato Sauce became a cherished meal, one they confidently prepared and thoroughly appreciated.

This chapter celebrates the joy of culinary growth and the magic of creating meals that inspire confidence and appreciation. As you and your young chefs prepare this delightful and wholesome dish together, may you savor the pride in mastering a culinary skill and the deliciousness that comes from enjoying a well-cooked zucchini noodle. Bon appétit!

Zucchini Noodles with Tomato Sauce:

Ingredients:
- 2 large zucchinis
- 1 can (14 ounces) diced tomatoes or tomato sauce
- 1 clove garlic, minced
- 1 tablespoon olive oil
- 1 teaspoon dried basil
- 1/2 teaspoon dried oregano
- Salt and pepper to taste
- Grated Parmesan cheese for topping (optional)

Instructions:

1. Wash the zucchinis and trim off the ends. Using a spiralizer or a vegetable peeler, create zucchini noodles by cutting the zucchinis into long, thin strips. If using a vegetable peeler, continue peeling the zucchinis lengthwise until you reach the seeds at the core. Discard the core or save it for other recipes.

2. In a saucepan over medium heat, add olive oil and minced garlic. Cook the garlic for a minute until it becomes fragrant.

3. Add the diced tomatoes or tomato sauce to the saucepan, and stir in the dried basil and oregano. Season with salt and pepper to taste.

4. Let the tomato sauce simmer for about 5-7 minutes, allowing the flavors to meld together.

5. In a separate non-stick skillet, sauté the zucchini noodles over medium heat for about 2-3 minutes until they are slightly softened but still have a bit of crunch.

6. Pour the tomato sauce over the zucchini noodles, and toss everything together until the noodles are well coated.

7. If you like, sprinkle some grated Parmesan cheese on top for added flavor.

8. Your Zucchini Noodles with Tomato Sauce are now ready to serve!

**Inspire young chefs to appreciate the art of making healthy choices in their Zucchini Noodles with Tomato Sauce, and to take pride in creating a garden of flavors on their culinary canvas. Cooking is an opportunity to express creativity and enjoy a delightful culinary journey. Happy swirling and culinary canvas creating!

27

Grilled Chicken Caesar Salad

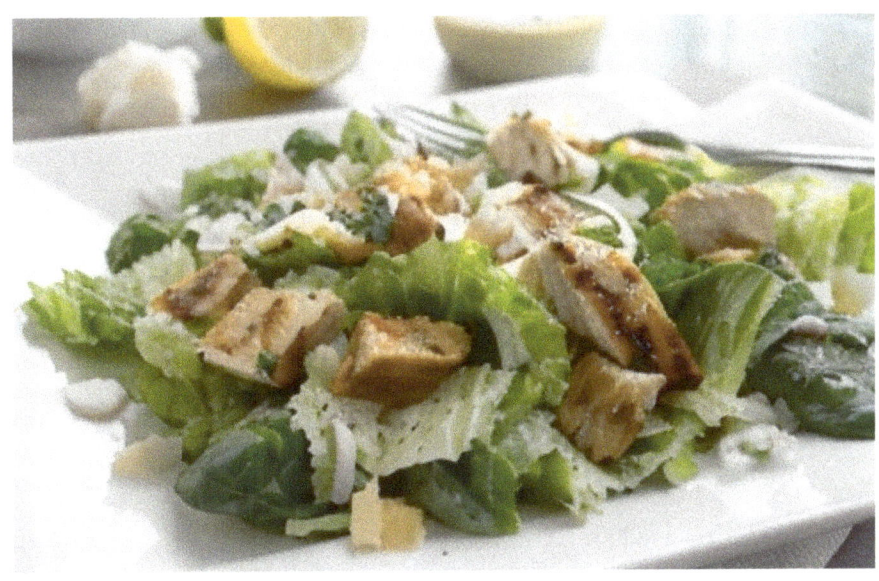

Grilled Chicken Caesar Salad

"*In every Caesar salad creation, you have the power to elevate greens with a touch of protein perfection. Embrace the balance of flavors with every bite!*" - *Papa True Ju*

In our kitchen, there's a tale of taste buds awakened and a delightful afternoon that led my sons to crave the flavorful Grilled Chicken Caesar Salad. This refreshing and satisfying meal holds a special place in their hearts, inspired by a warm afternoon before heading out for a day at the park, where their mother introduced them to this culinary delight.

One sunny day, before embarking on a family adventure to the park, their mother surprised them with a Grilled Chicken Caesar Salad. The tender grilled chicken, chosen for its savory and protein-rich qualities, became the centerpiece of this nourishing dish.

As they sat down to enjoy the salad, they watched with anticipation as she generously sprinkled crunchy croutons over fresh and crisp romaine lettuce. The croutons added a delightful texture and a satisfying crunch to the salad.

Next came the creamy Caesar dressing, expertly drizzled over the salad. The dressing, a harmonious blend of rich flavors, elevated the salad to a level of irresistible deliciousness.

With eager excitement, they took their first bites. The succulent grilled chicken, mingling with the crisp lettuce and zesty dressing, created a symphony of flavors that they couldn't get enough of.

From that moment on, Grilled Chicken Caesar Salad became a cherished meal, one they craved for its refreshing taste and nourishing goodness.

This chapter celebrates the joy of culinary discoveries and the magic of creating meals that become family favorites. As you and your young chefs prepare this refreshing and satisfying salad together, may you savor the taste of adventure and the deliciousness that comes from enjoying a Grilled Chicken Caesar Salad before heading out for a day of fun at the park. Bon appétit!

Grilled Chicken Caesar Salad:

Ingredients:
- 2 boneless, skinless chicken breasts
- Romaine lettuce, washed and torn into bite-sized pieces
- Caesar salad dressing (store-bought or homemade)
- Croutons
- Grated Parmesan cheese

Instructions:

1. Preheat your grill or stovetop grill pan over medium heat.

2. Season the chicken breasts with salt and pepper or any favorite seasoning of your choice.

3. Place the seasoned chicken breasts on the grill or grill pan.

4. Cook the chicken for about 5-7 minutes per side or until it reaches an internal temperature of 165°F (74°C) and is no longer pink in the center.

5. Once the chicken is done, remove it from the grill and let it rest for a moment before slicing.

6. In a large salad bowl, add the washed and torn romaine lettuce.

7. Drizzle Caesar salad dressing over the lettuce and toss until the lettuce is evenly coated with the dressing.

8. Add croutons and grated Parmesan cheese to the salad, and toss again to combine.

9. Slice the grilled chicken breasts into thin strips.

10. Arrange the sliced chicken on top of the Caesar salad.

11. Your Grilled Chicken Caesar Salad is now ready to enjoy!

**Inspire young chefs to appreciate the balance of flavors in their Grilled Chicken Caesar Salad, and to take pride in elevating greens with a touch of protein perfection. Cooking is an opportunity to create delicious and balanced masterpieces. Happy grilling and culinary creation!

28

Fruit Kabobs with Yogurt Dip

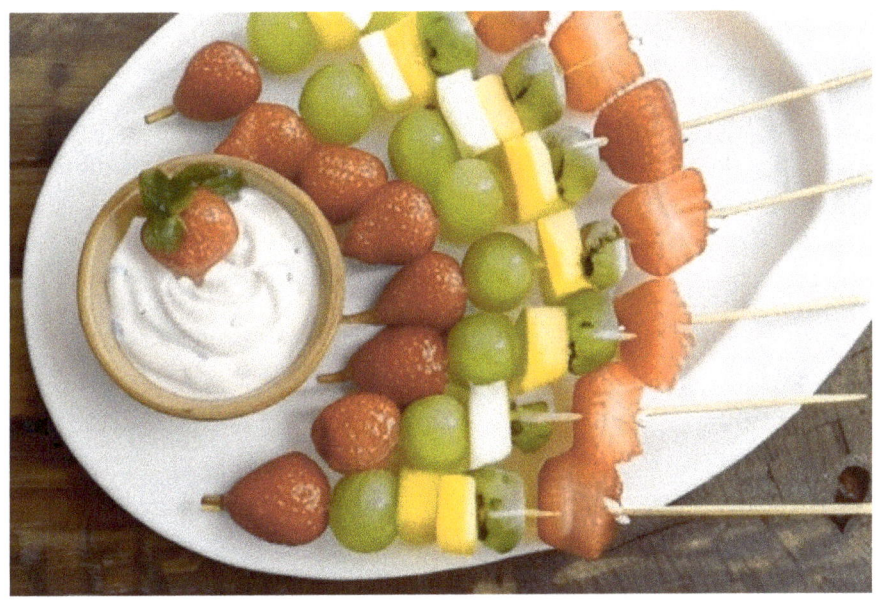

Fruit Kabobs with Yogurt Dip

"*In every fruit kabob, you have the power to weave a rainbow of flavors and create a culinary masterpiece. Embrace the magic of colors within your culinary creation!*" - Coach Rae

In our kitchen, there's a tale of curiosity and taste bud delights that led my sons to enjoy the fresh and vibrant flavors of Fruit Kabobs with Yogurt Dip. This refreshing and colorful meal holds a special place in their hearts, inspired by a television show that sparked their desire to try it out for themselves.

One day, they watched with fascination as a television show featured a colorful array of fresh fruits artfully arranged on skewers. The fruits, a medley of sweet and juicy goodness, became the star of the dish.

With excitement and determination, they decided to recreate the Fruit Kabobs with their twist. They carefully selected a variety of fresh fruits—luscious strawberries, succulent pineapple chunks, and sweet melon cubes. The fruits provided a burst of color and vitamins to the kabobs.

Next, they prepared a creamy yogurt dip—a perfect accompaniment to the fruity skewers. The yogurt dip, chosen for its velvety texture and tangy taste, added a refreshing contrast to the sweetness of the fruits.

As they skillfully threaded the fruits onto the skewers and presented them with a dollop of yogurt dip, their faces lit up with anticipation.

When they took their first bites, they were enchanted by the explosion of flavors and textures. The juicy fruits mingled with the creamy yogurt dip, creating a delightful symphony that they savored with joy.

From that moment on, Fruit Kabobs with Yogurt Dip became a cherished meal, one they enjoyed not just for its deliciousness but also for the joy of creating it themselves.

This chapter celebrates the joy of curiosity and the magic of creating meals that are both delightful to the eyes and the taste buds. As you and your young chefs prepare these refreshing and colorful fruit kabobs with yogurt dip together, may you savor the sense of adventure and the deliciousness that comes from enjoying a fun and wholesome meal. Bon appétit!

Fruit Kabobs with Yogurt Dip:

Ingredients:
- Assorted fresh fruits (e.g., strawberries, grapes, pineapple, melon, etc.)
- Wooden or metal skewers
- Yogurt dip (store-bought or homemade)

Instructions:

1. Wash and prepare the assorted fresh fruits. Cut them into bite-sized pieces, suitable for threading onto the skewers.

2. If you're using wooden skewers, soak them in water for about 30 minutes to prevent them from burning during use.

3. Take one fruit at a time and thread them onto the skewers in any desired pattern or combination.

4. Repeat the threading process with the remaining fruits and skewers.

5. Place the prepared fruit kabobs on a serving platter.

6. If you have a yogurt dip, transfer it to a small bowl or individual dipping cups.

7. Arrange the yogurt dip next to the fruit kabobs on the serving platter.

8. Your Fruit Kabobs with Yogurt Dip are now ready to serve!

**Inspire young chefs to appreciate the magic of colors in their Fruit Kabobs with Yogurt Dip, and to take pride in weaving a rainbow of flavors in their culinary masterpiece. Cooking is an opportunity to create delightful and colorful culinary creations. Happy threading and culinary magic!

29

Lentil Soup with Vegetables

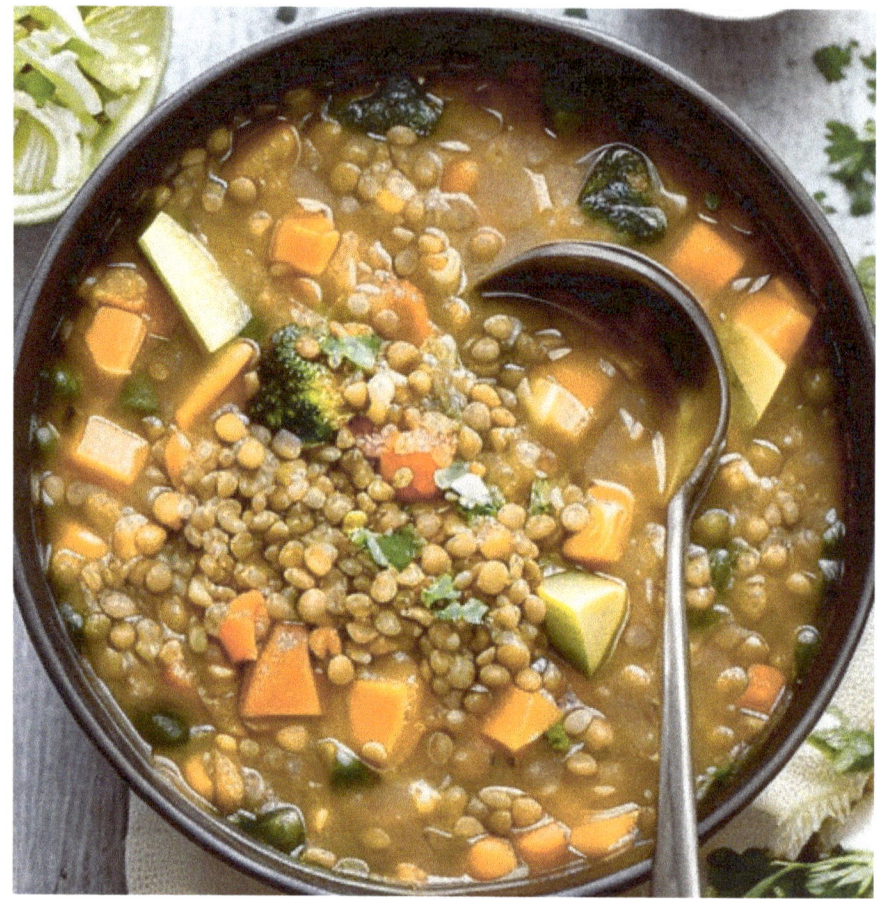

Lentil Soup with Vegetables

"*In every lentil soup, you have the power to simmer warmth and goodness and create a bowl of comfort. Embrace the art of nourishing flavors, and with every spoonful, feel the magnificence of your culinary creation!*" - Papa True Ju

In our kitchen, there's a tale of cultural heritage and a deep appreciation for the taste of Fresh Lentil Soup with Vegetables that my sons hold close to their hearts. This comforting and flavorful meal is not just a dish; it's a connection to their rich ancestry that they love to explore and savor.

LENTIL SOUP WITH VEGETABLES

As my sons grew older, they developed a keen interest in learning about their family's roots and the traditional dishes that have been passed down through generations. Lentil Soup with Vegetables is one such meal—a cherished part of their culture and heritage.

With enthusiasm, they discovered the secret to creating a hearty and wholesome Lentil Soup. They selected nutritious green lentils, chosen for their earthy flavor and rich protein content. The lentils became the heart of the soup, offering both taste and nourishment.

Next, they gathered fresh vegetables—carrots, celery, and onions. The vegetables not only added a delightful medley of colors but also enhanced the flavor and texture of the soup.

As they simmered the ingredients together, a delightful aroma filled the kitchen, reminding them of the comforting meals enjoyed by their ancestors.

The spices—warm and aromatic—came next. A pinch of cumin and a dash of paprika elevated the soup, adding a touch of warmth and depth to the flavors.

When they ladled the Lentil Soup with Vegetables into bowls and took their first spoonfuls, they were transported to a place of heritage and tradition. The soup, comforting and flavorful, warmed their hearts and souls.

From that moment on, Lentil Soup with Vegetables became a beloved meal, one that not only delighted their taste buds but also connected them to their rich ancestral roots.

This chapter celebrates the joy of embracing cultural heritage and the magic of creating meals that carry a sense of tradition and family history. As you and your young chefs prepare this comforting and flavorful Lentil Soup with Vegetables together, may you savor the connection to your heritage and the deliciousness that comes from enjoying a meal that is more than just food—it's a celebration of your ancestry. Bon appétit!

Lentil Soup with Vegetables:

Ingredients:
- 1 cup dried lentils (red or green), rinsed and sorted
- 4 cups vegetable broth or water
- 1 medium onion, chopped
- 2 carrots, peeled and diced
- 2 celery stalks, diced
- 2 cloves garlic, minced
- 1 bay leaf (optional)
- 1 teaspoon dried thyme
- 1 teaspoon ground cumin
- Salt and pepper to taste
- Olive oil for sautéing

Instructions:

1. In a large pot, heat a drizzle of olive oil over medium heat.

2. Add the chopped onion, diced carrots, and diced celery to the pot. Sauté the vegetables for about 5 minutes or until they begin to soften.

3. Stir in the minced garlic, dried thyme, and ground cumin, and sauté for another minute until the spices become fragrant.

4. Add the rinsed lentils and bay leaf (if using) to the pot, and stir everything together.

5. Pour in the vegetable broth or water, and bring the soup to a boil.

LENTIL SOUP WITH VEGETABLES

6. Once the soup is boiling, reduce the heat to low, cover the pot with a lid, and let it simmer for about 20-25 minutes or until the lentils and vegetables are tender.

7. Taste the soup and add salt and pepper to your liking.

8. Remove the bay leaf (if used) before serving.

9. Your Lentil Soup with Vegetables is now ready to enjoy!

**Inspire young chefs to appreciate the art of simmering warmth and goodness in their Lentil Soup with Vegetables, and to take pride in creating a bowl of comforting and nourishing flavors. Cooking is an opportunity to create culinary comfort and warmth. Happy simmering and culinary creation!

30

Baked Tilapia with a Side of Steamed Broccoli

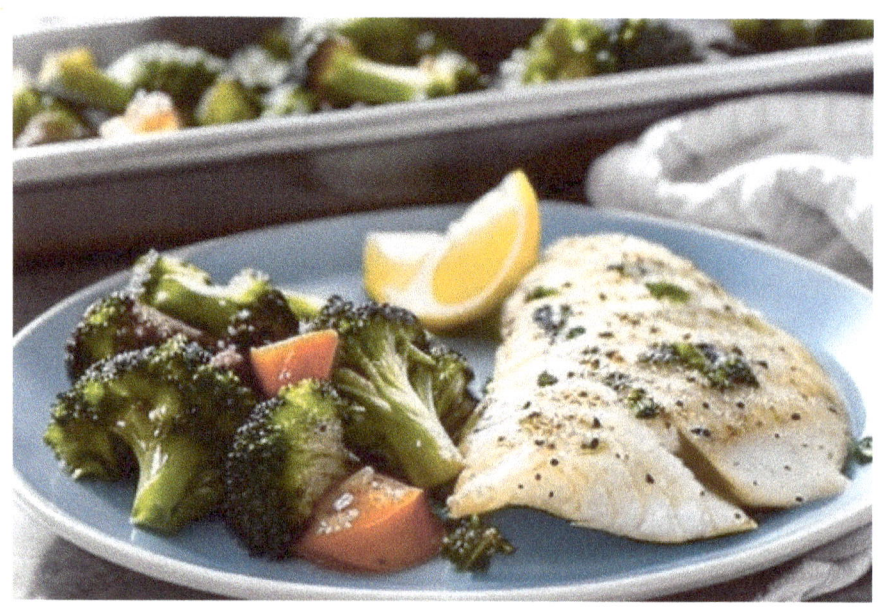

Baked Tilapia with a Side of Steamed Broccoli

"*In every tilapia fillet and steamed green delight, you have the power to plate health and freshness and create a culinary balance. Embrace*

BAKED TILAPIA WITH A SIDE OF STEAMED BROCCOLI

the harmony of tastes expertly baked into your culinary creation!" - Papa True Ju

In our kitchen, there's a tale of clean and rich-tasting foods that my sons adore, and the joy they found in the delicious Baked Tilapia with a Side of Steamed Broccoli—a meal that has delighted them from their very first bite.

From an early age, my sons developed a taste for clean and wholesome foods. They appreciated the purity of flavors and the goodness that comes from nourishing ingredients.

One day, they sat down to savor a meal that would become an instant favorite—the Baked Tilapia with a Side of Steamed Broccoli.

The star of the dish was the tender tilapia fillets, chosen for their mild and delicate taste. The tilapia, expertly seasoned with a hint of lemon and herbs, offered a rich-tasting and satisfying experience.

Alongside the tilapia, they enjoyed a side of vibrant steamed broccoli—a nutritious and flavorful addition to the meal.

As they took their first bites, their faces lit up with delight. The tilapia, perfectly baked to flaky perfection, paired wonderfully with the tender and bright green broccoli.

With each mouthful, they savored the clean and rich flavors that delighted their taste buds and satisfied their love for wholesome meals.

From that moment on, Baked Tilapia with a Side of Steamed Broccoli became a cherished meal, one that they requested time and again.

This chapter celebrates the joy of appreciating clean and rich-tasting foods and the magic of creating meals that bring delight and satisfaction. As you and your young chefs prepare this delicious Baked Tilapia with a Side of Steamed Broccoli together, may you savor the goodness of nourishing ingredients and the deliciousness that comes from enjoying a meal that delights both the palate and the heart. Bon appétit!

Baked Tilapia with a Side of Steamed Broccoli:

Ingredients:
- 2 tilapia fillets
- Lemon slices (optional)
- Salt and pepper to taste
- Olive oil for brushing
- 1 bunch of fresh broccoli, washed and trimmed

Instructions:

1. Preheat your oven to 400°F (200°C).

2. Pat dry the tilapia fillets with a paper towel to remove excess moisture.

3. Season the tilapia fillets with salt and pepper, and place them on a baking sheet lined with parchment paper.

4. If you like, place lemon slices on top of the tilapia fillets for added flavor.

5. Brush the tilapia fillets with a little olive oil to prevent sticking and enhance the taste.

6. Bake the tilapia in the preheated oven for about 12-15 minutes or until the fish is cooked through and flakes easily with a fork.

7. While the tilapia is baking, prepare the broccoli. Cut the broccoli into florets and place them in a steamer basket or a saucepan with a small amount

of water.

8. Steam the broccoli over medium heat for about 5-7 minutes or until it's tender-crisp.

9. Once the tilapia and broccoli are done, remove them from the oven and the steamer.

10. Your Baked Tilapia with a Side of Steamed Broccoli is now ready to serve!

**Inspire young chefs to appreciate the harmony of tastes in their Baked Tilapia with a Side of Steamed Broccoli, and to take pride in creating a balanced and healthy culinary plate. Cooking is an opportunity to plate freshness and balance. Happy baking, steaming, and culinary creativity!

31

Veggie-Loaded Pizza on Whole-Grain Crust

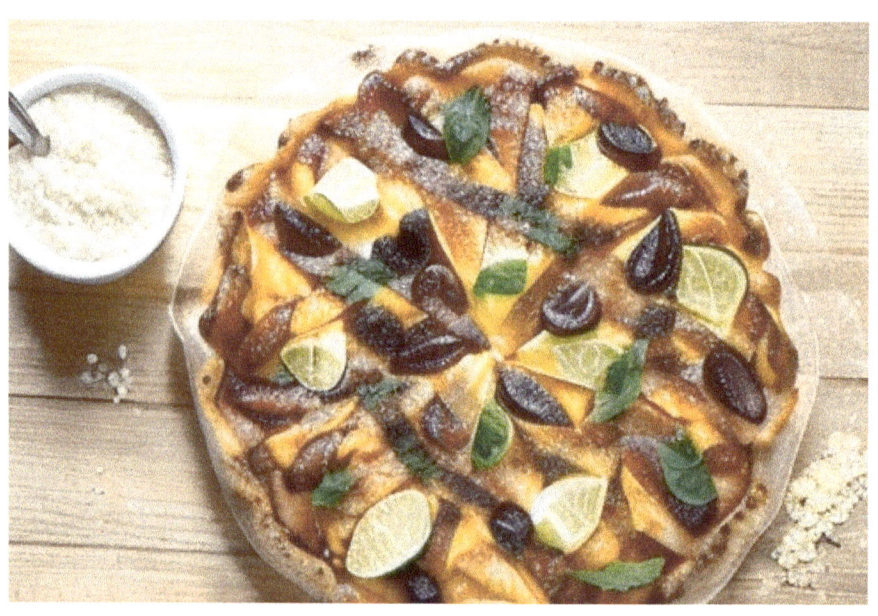

Veggie-Loaded Pizza on Whole-Grain Crust

"In every veggie-loaded slice, you have the power to create a garden of flavors and a culinary canvas. Embrace the art of nourishing choices,

VEGGIE-LOADED PIZZA ON WHOLE-GRAIN CRUST

and transfer this power into your daily activities!" - Papa True Ju

In our kitchen, there's a tale of pizza-loving boys who discovered the delightful world of Veggie-Loaded Pizza on Whole-Grain Crust—a meal that pleasantly surprised them from their very first bite, capturing their hearts with both taste and health benefits.

My sons have always had a soft spot for pizza, savoring every cheesy, saucy, and crispy bite. But one day, they embarked on a pizza adventure that would forever change their pizza preferences.

They gathered around the kitchen counter as we prepared the Veggie-Loaded Pizza. The foundation of this delicious creation was the whole-grain crust—a wise choice for its nutty flavor and rich source of fiber.

As they carefully spread a tangy tomato sauce over the crust, they knew that the journey to pizza perfection had just begun.

Next, they loaded the pizza with colorful and nutritious veggies—vibrant bell peppers, juicy cherry tomatoes, and tender spinach leaves. Each vegetable not only added a burst of color but also contributed essential vitamins and minerals.

A generous sprinkle of low-fat mozzarella cheese was the final touch, binding the flavors together and providing a delightful gooeyness they loved.

With eager anticipation, they watched as the pizza baked to golden perfection. The kitchen filled with a mouthwatering aroma that made their taste buds dance in excitement.

When they finally took their first bites, they were in awe of the deliciousness that greeted them. The whole-grain crust, packed with wholesome goodness, elevated the pizza to a new level of satisfaction.

With each slice, they relished the health benefits of their Veggie-Loaded Pizza, and their pizza-loving hearts found a new favorite that they couldn't get enough of.

From that moment on, Veggie-Loaded Pizza on Whole-Grain Crust became a cherished meal, one that delighted their taste buds and nourished their bodies with every delectable bite.

This chapter celebrates the joy of discovering the best of both worlds—the deliciousness of pizza and the health benefits of wholesome ingredients. As you and your young chefs prepare this Veggie-Loaded Pizza on Whole-Grain Crust together, may you savor the delightful flavors and the goodness of nourishing ingredients, creating a pizza experience that surprises and delights every time. Bon appétit!

Veggie-Loaded Pizza on Whole-Grain Crust:

Ingredients:
   - Whole-grain pizza crust (store-bought or homemade)
   - Tomato sauce or pizza sauce
   - Shredded mozzarella cheese (or any favorite cheese)
   - Assorted vegetables (e.g., bell peppers, mushrooms, onions, spinach, etc.), chopped or sliced
   - Optional toppings: olives, cherry tomatoes, or any other favorite toppings

Instructions:

1. Preheat your oven according to the pizza crust package instructions or your homemade crust recipe.

2. If using a store-bought whole-grain pizza crust, follow the package instructions for pre-baking (if needed).

VEGGIE-LOADED PIZZA ON WHOLE-GRAIN CRUST

3. Once the crust is pre-baked or ready for toppings, spread a layer of tomato or pizza sauce evenly over the crust, leaving a small border around the edges.

4. Sprinkle shredded mozzarella cheese (or any favorite cheese) over the sauce, covering the pizza evenly.

5. Now it's time to load up your pizza with colorful veggies! Spread the chopped or sliced vegetables over the cheese.

6. If you like, add any optional toppings, such as olives or cherry tomatoes, for added flavor and color.

7. Carefully transfer the topped pizza to a pizza stone, baking sheet, or pizza pan.

8. Bake the pizza in the preheated oven for about 10-15 minutes, or until the cheese is melted, bubbly, and slightly golden.

9. Once the pizza is done, remove it from the oven and let it cool for a moment.

10. Slice your Veggie-Loaded Pizza on Whole-Grain Crust and serve!

**Inspire young chefs to appreciate the art of nourishing choices in their Veggie-Loaded Pizza on Whole-Grain Crust, and to take pride in creating a colorful garden of flavors on their culinary canvas. Cooking is an opportunity to create delicious and nourishing masterpieces. Happy loading and culinary canvas creating!

32

Stuffed Mushrooms with Spinach and Cheese

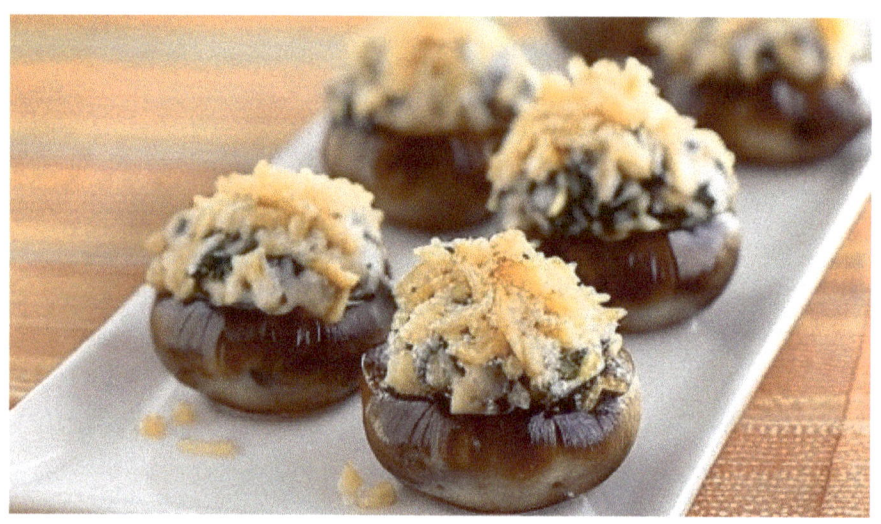

Stuffed Mushrooms with Spinach and Cheese

"*In every stuffed mushroom delight, you have the power to blend flavors and create a burst of goodness. Embrace the art of culinary creativity, and enjoy your meal with every bite!*"
- ***Coach Rae***

STUFFED MUSHROOMS WITH SPINACH AND CHEESE

In our kitchen, there's a tale of culinary exploration that broadened my sons' palates, introducing them to the wonderful world of Stuffed Mushrooms with Spinach and Cheese—a meal that they weren't too fond of at first but soon came to appreciate and savor.

One evening, we decided to embark on a journey of international flavors, and Stuffed Mushrooms with Spinach and Cheese was our destination.

As we gathered around the kitchen counter, my sons were a bit hesitant. Mushrooms weren't their favorite, and spinach was a new addition to their culinary repertoire.

With curiosity and open minds, they decided to take small bites of this intriguing dish.

The mushrooms, selected for their earthy and savory taste, served as delightful bite-sized vessels, waiting to be filled with a mixture of tender spinach and creamy cheese.

As they tasted the Stuffed Mushrooms, their palates were awakened to a medley of flavors they hadn't experienced before. The spinach added a gentle hint of freshness, while the cheese provided a rich and comforting creaminess.

With each bite, they discovered a harmony of tastes and textures that surprised them most delightfully.

As their journey of culinary exploration continued, they realized that trying new dishes allowed them to appreciate diverse flavors and expand their palate.

From that moment on, Stuffed Mushrooms with Spinach and Cheese became a meal they eagerly anticipated. The dish had become a gateway to international cuisine, encouraging them to embrace new flavors and culinary adventures.

This chapter celebrates the joy of trying new dishes and embracing diverse flavors from around the world. As you and your young chefs prepare Stuffed Mushrooms with Spinach and Cheese together, may you savor the delightful medley of flavors and the satisfaction of broadening your perspective of international cuisine. Bon appétit!

Stuffed Mushrooms with Spinach and Cheese:

Ingredients:
- 16-20 large white or cremini mushrooms, stems removed
- 1 cup fresh spinach, chopped
- 1/2 cup breadcrumbs
- 1/2 cup shredded mozzarella cheese (or any favorite cheese)
- 1/4 cup grated Parmesan cheese
- 2 cloves garlic, minced
- 2 tablespoons olive oil
- Salt and pepper to taste

Instructions:

1. Preheat your oven to 375°F (190°C).

2. Clean the mushrooms by gently wiping them with a damp cloth. Remove the stems and set them aside.

3. In a large bowl, combine the chopped spinach, breadcrumbs, shredded mozzarella cheese, grated Parmesan cheese, minced garlic, and olive oil. Mix everything until well combined.

4. Season the mixture with salt and pepper to taste.

STUFFED MUSHROOMS WITH SPINACH AND CHEESE

5. Take each mushroom cap and fill it with the spinach and cheese mixture, pressing it down gently to fit as much filling as possible.

6. Place the filled mushroom caps on a baking sheet lined with parchment paper.

7. Bake the stuffed mushrooms in the preheated oven for about 15-20 minutes, or until the mushrooms are tender and the cheese is melted and bubbly.

8. Once the stuffed mushrooms are done, remove them from the oven and let them cool for a moment.

9. Your Stuffed Mushrooms with Spinach and Cheese are now ready to serve!

**Inspire young chefs to appreciate the art of culinary creativity in their Stuffed Mushrooms with Spinach and Cheese, and to take pride in blending flavors to create a burst of goodness. Cooking is an opportunity to express creativity and enjoy a delightful culinary journey. Happy stuffing and culinary creativity!

33

Fruit and Yogurt Popsicles

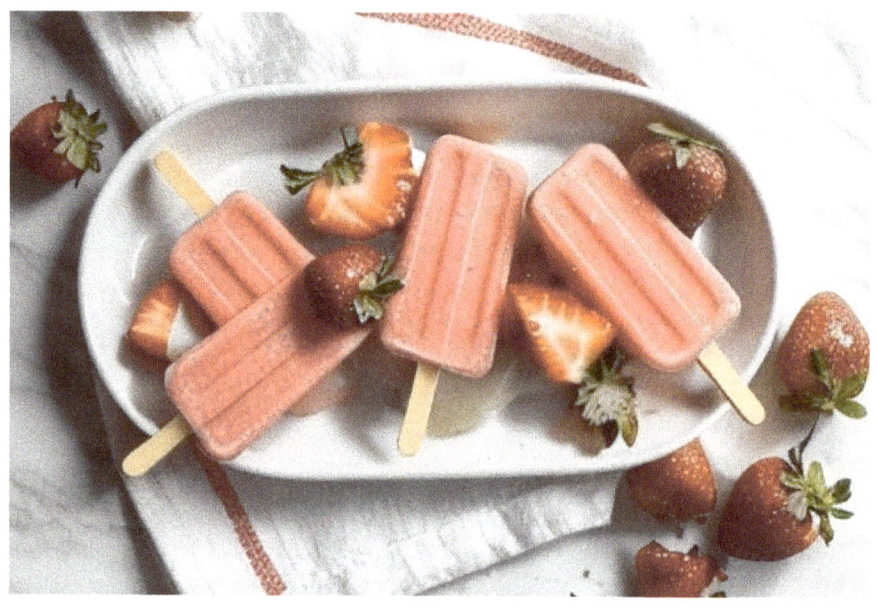

Fruit and Yogurt Popsicles

"*In every frozen delight, you have the power to blend flavors and create a symphony of sweetness. Embrace the art of healthy treats, and give your heart another reason to beat!*"
- *Papa True Ju*

FRUIT AND YOGURT POPSICLES

In our kitchen, there's a tale of summertime delights and the joy of crafting our very own Fruit and Yogurt Popsicles—a treat that brings smiles to my sons' faces with every lick.

As the days grew warmer, my sons eagerly awaited the moment we would create these delightful frozen treats.

The foundation of these popsicles was creamy yogurt—a choice made for its refreshing and smooth texture, perfect for a cool summer treat.

With excitement, they selected an array of vibrant and juicy fruits—ripe strawberries, succulent blueberries, and sweet mango slices. Each fruit added its burst of flavor and natural sweetness to the popsicles.

Carefully layering the fruit with the yogurt in popsicle molds, they created a beautiful mosaic of colors and flavors.

As they placed the molds in the freezer, anticipation filled the air. They knew that soon, their hard work would be rewarded with a frozen delight.

When the time came to taste their Fruit and Yogurt Popsicles, their faces lit up with delight. The cool and creamy yogurt paired harmoniously with the refreshing sweetness of the fruits.

With each lick, they savored the delightful combination of flavors, knowing that they had crafted something truly special.

From that moment on, Fruit and Yogurt Popsicles became a summertime favorite—a treat that they not only loved to consume but also enjoyed preparing.

This chapter celebrates the joy of summertime and the delight of crafting your very own frozen creations. As you and your young chefs prepare Fruit and Yogurt Popsicles together, may you savor the refreshing goodness of yogurt and the vibrant sweetness of fresh fruits, creating frozen delights that bring joy and smiles on warm summer days. Bon appétit!

Fruit and Yogurt Popsicles:

Ingredients:
- Assorted fresh fruits (e.g., berries, mango, kiwi, etc.), washed and chopped
- Greek yogurt or any favorite yogurt
- Honey or maple syrup (optional, for added sweetness)
- Popsicle molds or small paper cups
- Popsicle sticks

Instructions:

1. Prepare the assorted fresh fruits by washing them and chopping them into bite-sized pieces.

2. In a bowl, mix the chopped fruits with Greek yogurt until they are well coated. If you like, add a drizzle of honey or maple syrup for added sweetness, but this step is optional, as the natural sweetness of the fruits and yogurt can be delicious on its own.

3. Carefully spoon the fruit and yogurt mixture into the popsicle molds or small paper cups, making sure to fill them to the top.

4. Insert a popsicle stick into the center of each mold or cup, ensuring that the stick stands upright in the middle.

5. Place the popsicle molds or cups in the freezer, and let them freeze for at least 4-6 hours or until they are completely frozen.

6. Once the popsicles are frozen, remove them from the freezer.

7. If using popsicle molds, carefully unmold the popsicles by running warm water over the molds for a few seconds. If using paper cups, gently tear away the paper.

8. Your Fruit and Yogurt Popsicles are now ready to enjoy!

**Inspire young chefs to appreciate the art of healthy treats in their Fruit and Yogurt Popsicles, and to take pride in creating a symphony of sweetness with blended flavors. Cooking is an opportunity to create delightful and healthy frozen masterpieces. Happy freezing and culinary creativity!

34

Teriyaki Tofu with Rice and Steamed Veggies

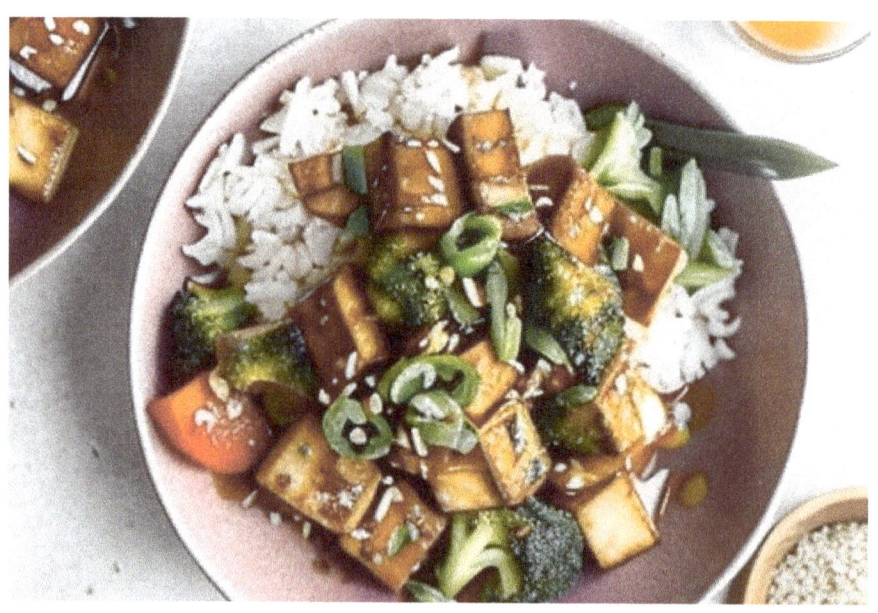

Teriyaki Tofu with Rice and Steamed Veggies

"*In every teriyaki tofu bowl, you have the power to blend tastes and create an Asian-inspired masterpiece. Embrace the harmony*

TERIYAKI TOFU WITH RICE AND STEAMED VEGGIES

of flavors, and with every bite, taste the success of your culinary creation!" - Coach Rae

In our kitchen, there's a heartwarming tale of teamwork and culinary triumph as my sons joyfully work together to prepare and cook Teriyaki Tofu with Rice and Steamed Veggies—a meal that delights the entire family with its flavors and the love put into its creation.

It all began one evening when my sons decided to take charge of dinner preparations. They wanted to create a meal that was not only delicious but also nutritious, pleasing everyone at the table.

Teriyaki Tofu with Rice and Steamed Veggies became their culinary adventure of choice.

They gathered around the kitchen counter, each with a role to play. One diligently prepared the tofu, pressing it to remove excess water, and cutting it into perfect bite-sized pieces. The tofu was their protein choice, known for its versatility and ability to soak up the savory teriyaki sauce.

Another was in charge of the vegetables—colorful bell peppers, tender broccoli florets, and crisp sugar snap peas. These veggies were chosen for their vibrant colors, enticing crunch, and nutritional benefits.

With smiles and laughter, they collaborated in making the teriyaki sauce—a blend of soy sauce, ginger, garlic, and a hint of sweetness that would infuse the tofu and veggies with delightful Asian flavors.

As they sautéed the tofu and veggies in the sauce, the kitchen filled with a mouthwatering aroma that made everyone's stomach rumble in anticipation.

When it was time to serve, they carefully arranged the Teriyaki Tofu, Rice, and Steamed Veggies on each plate, creating a beautiful and appetizing meal.

As the family gathered around the dinner table, they knew that this meal was something special. The flavors were a symphony of umami, sweetness, and freshness that delighted every taste bud.

From that moment on, Teriyaki Tofu with Rice and Steamed Veggies became a cherished family favorite—a meal that showcased their teamwork and culinary prowess, leaving everyone at the table satisfied and smiling.

This chapter celebrates the joy of working together in the kitchen and the satisfaction of creating a meal that brings happiness to the entire family. As you and your young chefs prepare Teriyaki Tofu with Rice and Steamed Veggies together, may you savor the delicious flavors and the heartwarming spirit of teamwork, creating a culinary masterpiece that unites your family with love and joy. Bon appétit!

Teriyaki Tofu with Rice and Steamed Veggies:

Ingredients:
   - 1 block of firm tofu, drained and cubed
   - Teriyaki sauce (store-bought or homemade)
   - 1 cup uncooked rice
   - Assorted vegetables (e.g., broccoli, carrots, bell peppers, etc.), washed and chopped
   - Soy sauce (optional, for seasoning)
   - Sesame seeds and green onions for garnish (optional)

Instructions:

1. Prepare the tofu by draining it and cutting it into bite-sized cubes.

2. Marinate the tofu cubes in teriyaki sauce, making sure they are well coated. Let it marinate for about 15-20 minutes to absorb the flavors.

TERIYAKI TOFU WITH RICE AND STEAMED VEGGIES

3. While the tofu is marinating, cook the rice according to package instructions or using your preferred method.

4. In a separate saucepan or steamer, steam the chopped vegetables until they are tender-crisp. If desired, season the steamed veggies with a dash of soy sauce for added flavor.

5. In a non-stick skillet over medium heat, cook the marinated tofu cubes until they are browned and slightly crispy on all sides.

6. Once the tofu is done, remove it from the skillet and set it aside.

7. Now it's time to assemble the meal. In each serving bowl or plate, layer a bed of cooked rice, followed by the teriyaki tofu cubes, and the steamed vegetables.

8. If you like, sprinkle sesame seeds and chopped green onions on top for a delightful garnish.

9. Your Teriyaki Tofu with Rice and Steamed Veggies is now ready to enjoy!

35

Egg Salad Lettuce Cups

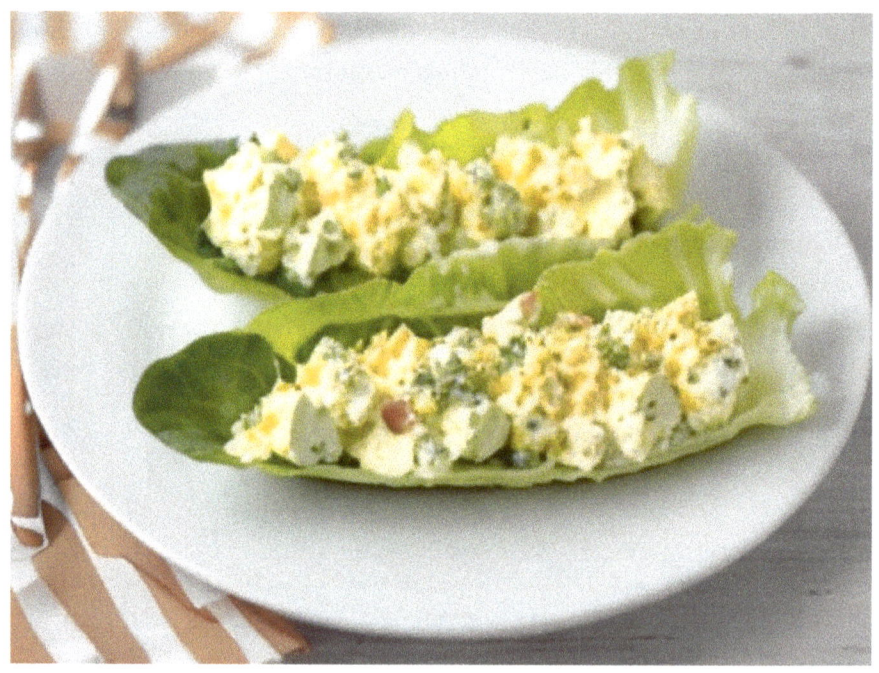

Egg Salad Lettuce Cups

"*In every egg salad creation, you have the power to balance tastes and create a wholesome delight. Embrace the art of fresh choices and*

completing a meaningful goal!"
- *Papa True Ju*

In our kitchen, there's a tale of culinary curiosity and the discovery of a unique and delightful meal—Egg Salad Lettuce Cups—a dish that initially seemed strange to my sons but quickly became a favorite for its simplicity and surprising deliciousness.

One day, as we were brainstorming new recipes, my sons spotted a picture of Egg Salad Lettuce Cups in a cookbook. Their curiosity piqued, and they couldn't help but wonder what this intriguing dish tasted like.

As they prepared the Egg Salad, they carefully boiled the eggs to perfection. Eggs were chosen for their versatility and nutrient-rich profile, offering a delicious source of protein.

With a gentle touch, they mixed the eggs with creamy mayonnaise, tangy mustard, and a sprinkle of chives, creating a delectable egg salad mixture.

Then came the moment of truth—the lettuce cups. They took fresh, crisp lettuce leaves, using them as a unique and nutritious alternative to bread or tortilla wraps.

With a mixture of excitement and hesitation, they scooped the Egg Salad into the lettuce cups, unsure of what to expect.

As they took their first bite, their faces lit up with surprise and delight. The crunch of the lettuce perfectly complemented the creamy egg salad filling, creating a refreshing and satisfying combination of textures and flavors.

What initially seemed strange had quickly become one of the more unique and beloved meals they had tried.

From that moment on, Egg Salad Lettuce Cups became a fun and wholesome meal they enjoyed preparing and eating. They loved how easy it was to customize the flavors by adding their favorite herbs and seasonings.

This chapter celebrates the joy of culinary curiosity and the thrill of discovering delightful flavors in unexpected combinations. As you and your young chefs prepare Egg Salad Lettuce Cups together, may you embrace the spirit of adventure and relish in the delightful surprise of a unique and delicious meal. Bon appétit!

Egg Salad Lettuce Cups:

Ingredients:
  - 4 hard-boiled eggs, peeled and chopped
  - 1/4 cup mayonnaise
  - 1 teaspoon Dijon mustard (optional, for added flavor)
  - Salt and pepper to taste
  - Lettuce leaves (e.g., romaine, butter lettuce, etc.) for serving
  - Optional toppings: sliced cherry tomatoes, cucumber, or any other favorite veggies

Instructions:

1. In a mixing bowl, combine the chopped hard-boiled eggs with mayonnaise and Dijon mustard (if using).

2. Stir the mixture until the eggs are well coated with the creamy dressing.

3. Season the egg salad with salt and pepper to taste.

4. Wash and prepare the lettuce leaves, ensuring they are dry and ready for serving.

EGG SALAD LETTUCE CUPS

5. To assemble the egg salad lettuce cups, take one lettuce leaf and spoon a portion of the egg salad onto the center of the leaf.

6. If you like, add optional toppings, such as sliced cherry tomatoes, cucumber, or any other favorite veggies on top of the egg salad for added freshness and flavor.

7. Fold the lettuce leaf gently over the egg salad to create a cup-like shape.

8. Repeat the process with the remaining lettuce leaves and egg salad.

9. Your Egg Salad Lettuce Cups are now ready to enjoy!

**Inspire young chefs to appreciate the art of fresh choices in their Egg Salad Lettuce Cups, and to take pride in creating a wholesome and balanced culinary delight. Cooking is an opportunity to create fresh and delightful masterpieces. Happy assembling and culinary creativity!

36

Cucumber and Cream Cheese Sandwiches

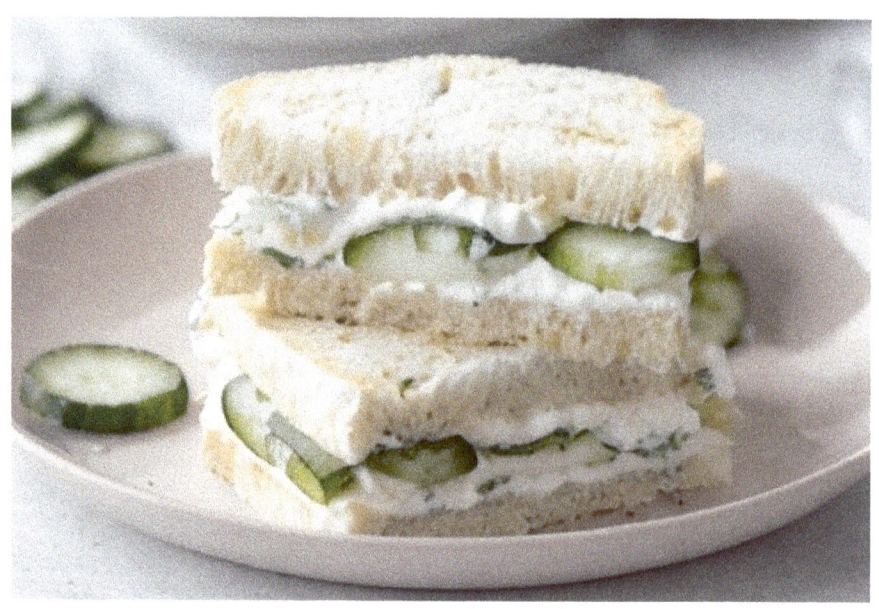

Cucumber and Cream Cheese Sandwiches

"*In every cucumber sandwich, you have the power to layer goodness and create a light and refreshing delight. Embrace the art of sandwich*

CUCUMBER AND CREAM CHEESE SANDWICHES

crafting, one loaf of bread at a time!"
- ***Divine Family Unit***

In our kitchen, there's a tale of delightful surprises and quick pick-me-ups before intense workouts—Cucumber and Cream Cheese Sandwiches—a surprisingly delicious meal that my sons enjoy.

It all began on a sunny afternoon when my sons were gearing up for a challenging sports practice. They needed a quick, energizing snack to fuel their bodies and keep them going strong.

In search of something refreshing and light, they discovered the magic of Cucumber and Cream Cheese Sandwiches.

They carefully sliced fresh cucumbers, choosing them for their crispness and hydrating properties, perfect for replenishing their energy.

Then came the cream cheese—a smooth and creamy spread that they adore. It provided the right balance of creaminess to complement the crunch of the cucumbers.

With a sprinkle of dill and a pinch of salt, they added a burst of flavor that elevated the simple sandwich to a delightful treat.

As they took their first bite, they were pleasantly surprised by the burst of freshness and creaminess. The combination of flavors and textures was perfect for a quick pick-me-up before their intense workout.

From that moment on, Cucumber and Cream Cheese Sandwiches became a staple in their pre-workout routine—a treat that kept them energized and ready to take on any challenge.

This chapter celebrates the joy of simple pleasures and the magic of surprising flavors. As you and your young chefs prepare Cucumber and Cream Cheese Sandwiches together, may you savor the refreshing taste and the delight of discovering unexpected culinary delights. Bon appétit!

Cucumber and Cream Cheese Sandwiches:

Ingredients:
- Sliced bread (white, whole-grain, or any favorite type)
- Cream cheese (regular or flavored)
- Cucumber, washed and thinly sliced
- Optional: Fresh dill, chives, or any favorite herbs for added flavor

Instructions:

1. Lay out the slices of bread on a clean work surface.

2. Spread a generous layer of cream cheese on one side of each bread slice. You can use regular cream cheese or try flavored cream cheese for extra taste.

3. Take a few cucumber slices and arrange them on top of the cream cheese layer on one bread slice.

4. If you like, sprinkle fresh dill, chives, or any favorite herbs on top of the cucumber for added flavor.

5. Carefully place the second bread slice on top of the cucumber slices, cream cheese side down, to form a sandwich.

6. Press the sandwich together gently to ensure the filling stays in place.

7. Using a sharp knife, cut off the crusts from the edges of the sandwich if desired.

8. Slice the sandwich diagonally to create two triangular halves or vertically to create rectangular halves.

9. Your Cucumber and Cream Cheese Sandwiches are now ready to serve!

**Inspire young chefs to appreciate the art of sandwich crafting in their Cucumber and Cream Cheese Sandwiches, and to take pride in layering goodness to create a light and refreshing culinary delight. Cooking is an opportunity to create delightful and refreshing masterpieces. Happy sandwich crafting and culinary creativity!

37

Quinoa-Stuffed Bell Peppers

QUINOA-STUFFED BELL PEPPERS

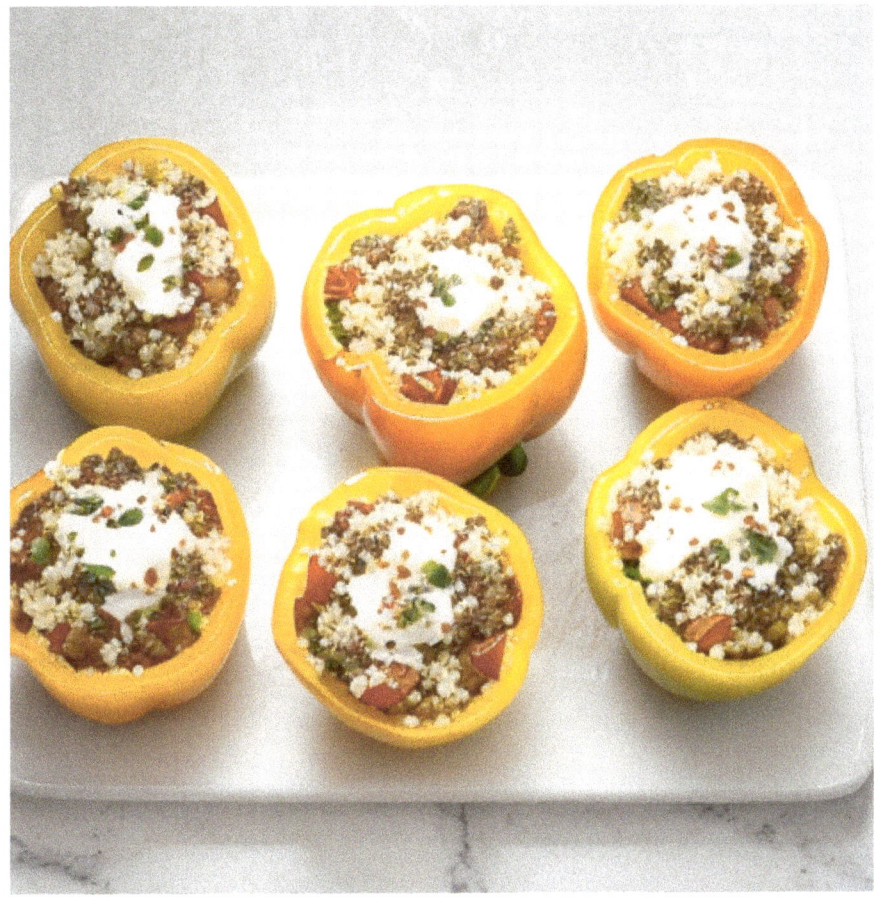

Quinoa-Stuffed Bell Peppers

"*In every quinoa-stuffed bell pepper, you have the power to create a wholesome and colorful meal. Embrace the art of nutritious stuffing, and share the love of your culinary creation with others!*" - Coach Rae

In our kitchen, there's a tale of a delightful twist on a family favorite that left my sons thrilled and eager for more—Quinoa-Stuffed Bell Peppers—a dish that has been a hit with them from the very first bite.

The story began when my sons tasted stuffed bell peppers for the first time at their uncle's house. They loved the flavorful combination of tender bell peppers filled with a hearty and savory filling.

Inspired by their enthusiasm, I decided to put my delicious twist on this beloved dish—Quinoa-Stuffed Bell Peppers.

Quinoa took center stage as the star ingredient. We chose it for its nutty flavor and rich nutritional profile, providing a good source of protein and essential vitamins.

As we prepared the quinoa, we sautéed lean ground turkey, adding a wholesome and lean protein to the mix.

To enhance the flavors further, we mixed in a medley of fresh vegetables, including sweet corn, diced tomatoes, and vibrant green onions.

As the filling simmered, the kitchen was filled with a tantalizing aroma that left my sons eagerly waiting to taste the final creation.

Once the quinoa filling was ready, we carefully stuffed the vibrant bell peppers, using them as delightful and nutritious vessels.

With a sprinkle of cheese on top, we baked the stuffed bell peppers to perfection, allowing the flavors to meld and the cheese to melt into a golden crust.

The moment of truth came when my sons took their first bite of the Quinoa-Stuffed Bell Peppers. Their faces lit up with delight as they discovered the wonderful fusion of flavors and the wholesome goodness packed into each bite.

From that day on, Quinoa-Stuffed Bell Peppers have been a welcomed surprise and a family favorite. It's a dish that brings joy to our table, celebrating the love for good food and the thrill of discovering new and delicious twists on familiar classics.

This chapter celebrates the joy of culinary exploration and the pleasure of sharing family favorites with a delightful twist. As you and your young chefs prepare Quinoa-Stuffed Bell Peppers together, may you relish in the excitement of discovering delightful new flavors and creating lasting memories in the heart of your home. Bon appétit!

Quinoa-Stuffed Bell Peppers:

Ingredients:
- 4 large bell peppers (any color), washed and halved
- 1 cup quinoa, rinsed
- 2 cups vegetable broth or water
- 1 can (15 ounces) black beans, drained and rinsed
- 1 cup diced tomatoes (canned or fresh)
- 1 cup corn kernels (canned, frozen, or fresh)
- 1 teaspoon ground cumin
- 1 teaspoon chili powder (optional, for added heat)
- Salt and pepper to taste
- Shredded cheese (cheddar, mozzarella, or any favorite cheese) for topping (optional)
- Fresh cilantro or parsley for garnish (optional)

Instructions:

1. Preheat your oven to 375°F (190°C).

2. Cut the bell peppers in half vertically, removing the seeds and membranes. This will create a cavity for the quinoa stuffing.

3. In a saucepan, combine the quinoa and vegetable broth or water. Bring it to a boil, then reduce the heat to low, cover the saucepan with a lid, and

let the quinoa simmer for about 15-20 minutes or until it's cooked and the liquid is absorbed.

4. In a large mixing bowl, combine the cooked quinoa, black beans, diced tomatoes, corn kernels, ground cumin, and chili powder (if using).

5. Season the quinoa mixture with salt and pepper to taste, and stir everything together until it's well-mixed.

6. Carefully stuff each bell pepper half with the quinoa mixture, pressing it down gently to pack in as much filling as possible.

7. If you like, sprinkle shredded cheese on top of each stuffed pepper for added flavor and texture.

8. Place the stuffed bell peppers on a baking sheet lined with parchment paper.

9. Bake the stuffed bell peppers in the preheated oven for about 20-25 minutes or until the peppers are tender and the filling is heated through.

10. Once the stuffed bell peppers are done, remove them from the oven and let them cool for a moment.

11. If desired, garnish the stuffed peppers with fresh cilantro or parsley before serving.

12. Your Quinoa-Stuffed Bell Peppers are now ready to enjoy!

**Inspire young chefs to appreciate the art of nutritious stuffing in their Quinoa-Stuffed Bell Peppers, and to take pride in creating a wholesome and colorful culinary masterpiece. Cooking is an opportunity to create nutritious and delightful meals. Happy stuffing and culinary creativity!

38

Veggie and Cheese Frittata

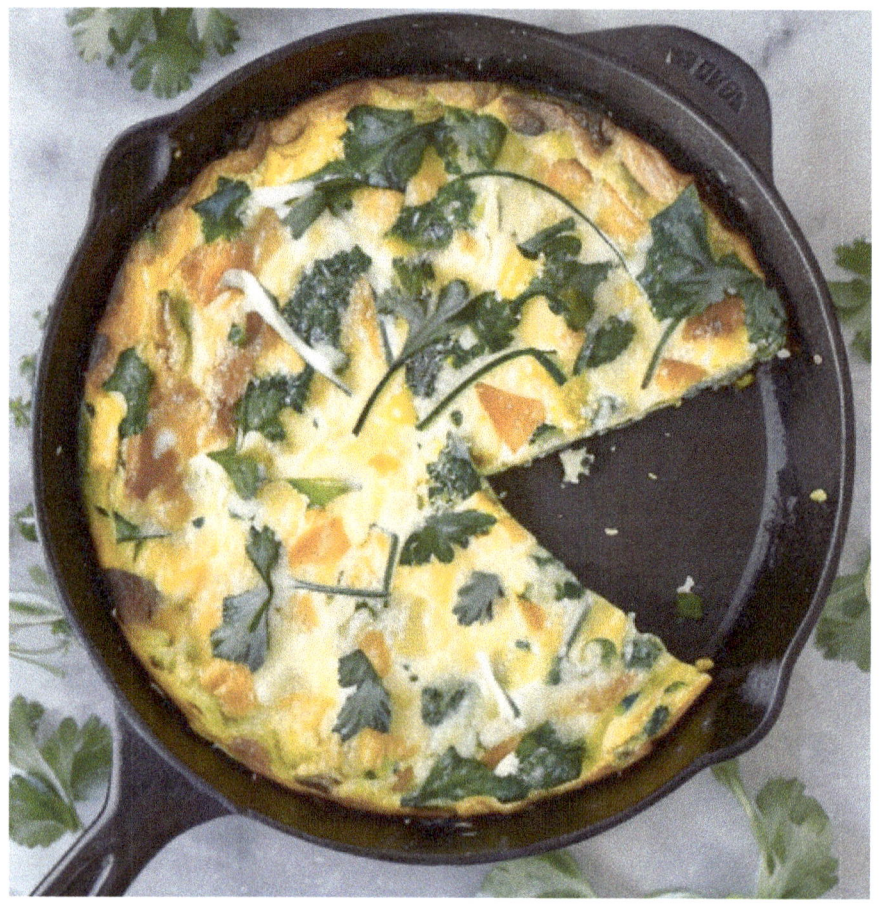

Veggie and Cheese Frittata

"*In every frittata creation, you have the power to blend flavors and create a delightful masterpiece. Embrace the art of frittata making, and share your culinary creation with friends and loved ones!*" - **Divine Family Unit**

In our kitchen, there's a tale of pure excitement and culinary discovery—Veggie and Cheese Frittata—a dish that left my sons ecstatic from the very first bite.

The story began on a bright Sunday morning when my sons woke up to the enticing aroma of a frittata cooking in the oven.

As they hurried to the kitchen, they found me preparing a medley of fresh vegetables—colorful bell peppers, tender spinach, and vibrant cherry tomatoes.

They watched in awe as I cracked open eggs, whisking them to fluffy perfection. The eggs symbolized a blank canvas, ready to be adorned with the vibrant colors and flavors of the vegetables.

We carefully layered the vegetables in a hot skillet, allowing them to gently sauté until they were tender and bursting with flavor.

With a sprinkle of cheese on top, we poured the whipped eggs over the vegetables, creating a beautiful mosaic of colors and textures.

As the frittata cooked, the kitchen was filled with a mouthwatering aroma that made my sons impatient with anticipation.

Finally, the moment they had been waiting for arrived as we took the frittata out of the oven. The golden edges and fluffy center made it an irresistible sight.

With eager anticipation, my sons took their first bite of the Veggie and Cheese Frittata. Their faces lit up with pure joy as they tasted the harmony of flavors—a delightful dance of vegetables and creamy cheese, perfectly complemented by the fluffy eggs.

From that day on, Veggie and Cheese Frittata has been a breakfast favorite, bringing excitement and joy to our mornings.

This chapter celebrates the thrill of discovering a delicious and nutritious breakfast option that leaves young chefs eager to create culinary masterpieces. As you and your young chefs prepare Veggie and Cheese Frittata together, may you share in the excitement of cooking and the joy of savoring wholesome flavors. Bon appétit!

Veggie and Cheese Frittata:

Ingredients:
- 6 large eggs
- 1/4 cup milk (regular or plant-based)
- 1 cup diced vegetables (e.g., bell peppers, onions, spinach, etc.)
- 1/2 cup shredded cheese (cheddar, mozzarella, or any favorite cheese)
- Salt and pepper to taste
- 1 tablespoon olive oil

Instructions:

1. Preheat your oven to 375°F (190°C).

2. In a mixing bowl, crack the eggs and whisk them together with the milk until well combined. Season with salt and pepper.

3. Heat the olive oil in an oven-safe skillet over medium heat.

4. Add the diced vegetables to the skillet and sauté them until they are tender. You can use any vegetables you like or have on hand.

5. Once the vegetables are cooked, spread them out evenly in the skillet.

6. Pour the whisked egg mixture over the sautéed vegetables, making sure the vegetables are evenly distributed throughout the eggs.

7. Sprinkle the shredded cheese on top of the egg and vegetable mixture.

VEGGIE AND CHEESE FRITTATA

8. Let the frittata cook on the stovetop for about 2-3 minutes or until the edges start to set.

9. Transfer the skillet to the preheated oven and bake the frittata for about 12-15 minutes or until it's fully set and the cheese is melted and bubbly.

10. Once the frittata is done, remove the skillet from the oven (be careful, it will be hot!).

11. Let the frittata cool for a moment before slicing it into wedges or squares.

12. Your Veggie and Cheese Frittata is now ready to serve!

**Inspire young chefs to appreciate the art of frittata making in their Veggie and Cheese Frittata, and to take pride in blending flavors to create a delightful culinary masterpiece. Cooking is an opportunity to create delicious and savory masterpieces. Happy frittata making and culinary creativity!

39

Baked Chicken Tenders with Sweet Potato Wedges

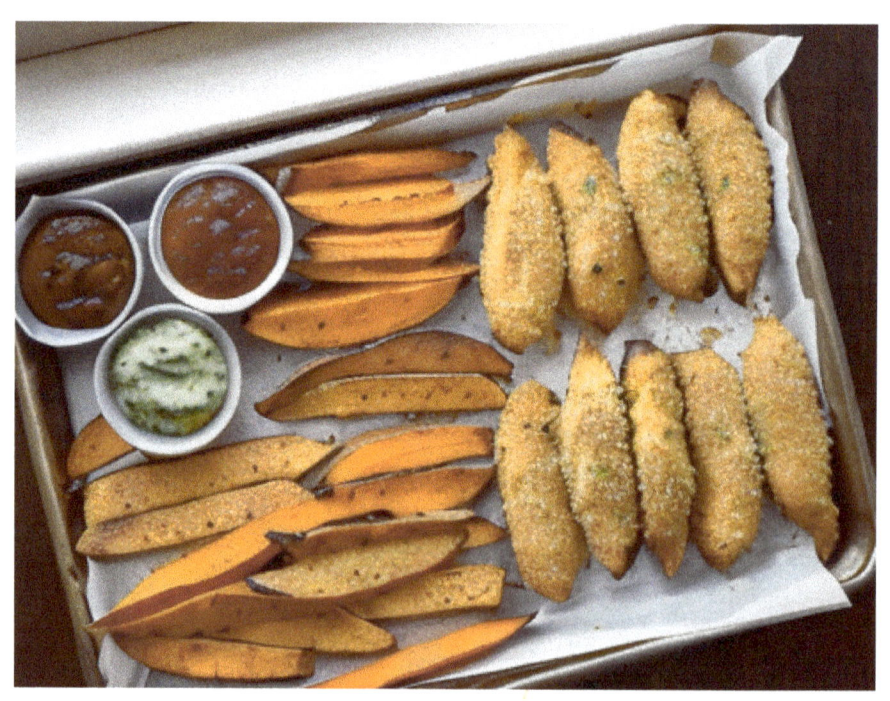

Baked Chicken Tenders with Sweet Potato Wedges

BAKED CHICKEN TENDERS WITH SWEET POTATO WEDGES

"*In every baked chicken tender and sweet potato wedge, you have the power to make a wholesome and balanced meal. Embrace the art of healthy cooking, and enjoy the success of your culinary creation!*" - Papa True Ju

The story of Baked Chicken Tenders with Sweet Potato Wedges is one of heartfelt delight—a meal personally requested by my sons to be featured in this very cookbook.

It all started on a cozy Sunday evening when my sons were craving a dish that was both satisfying and wholesome. As I gathered ingredients in the kitchen, they eagerly watched, their anticipation growing.

We began by preparing succulent chicken tenders, marinating them in a blend of savory herbs and spices. These tender chicken strips were carefully coated in a crispy whole-grain breadcrumb mixture, promising a delightful crunch with every bite.

While the chicken baked to golden perfection, we turned our attention to sweet potatoes—a family favorite. My sons loved the vibrant orange color and the natural sweetness of these nutrient-rich root vegetables.

We sliced the sweet potatoes into wedges, drizzled them with a hint of olive oil, and seasoned them with a pinch of sea salt and a sprinkle of aromatic herbs.

As the chicken tenders and sweet potato wedges baked side by side in the oven, the mouthwatering aroma filled our home, heightening our excitement for the delightful dinner ahead.

When the timer finally chimed, we couldn't wait to taste the result of our culinary collaboration. The tender chicken tenders were a burst of flavor, while the sweet potato wedges offered the perfect balance of sweetness and earthiness.

With wide smiles and full hearts, my sons declared this meal an absolute winner. They requested that this dish be featured in our cookbook, knowing that other young chefs and their families would find joy in preparing and savoring it too.

And so, in Chapter 39, we celebrate the power of shared moments in the kitchen—of creating dishes that bring pure delight and satisfaction. As you and your young chefs embark on preparing Baked Chicken Tenders with Sweet Potato Wedges, may your hearts be filled with the warmth of family-inspired meals and the joy of culinary exploration. Enjoy every flavorful bite!

Baked Chicken Tenders with Sweet Potato Wedges:

Ingredients:
- 1 pound chicken tenders (about 8-10 pieces)
- 2 large sweet potatoes, washed and cut into wedges
- 1/4 cup all-purpose flour (or any preferred flour)
- 1 teaspoon paprika
- 1/2 teaspoon garlic powder
- 1/2 teaspoon onion powder
- Salt and pepper to taste
- 2 tablespoons olive oil
- Cooking spray or olive oil spray

Instructions:

1. Preheat your oven to 425°F (220°C).

2. Prepare a baking sheet by lining it with parchment paper or lightly greasing it with cooking spray.

BAKED CHICKEN TENDERS WITH SWEET POTATO WEDGES

3. In a shallow dish or bowl, combine the flour, paprika, garlic powder, onion powder, salt, and pepper. Mix the dry ingredients.

4. Dredge each chicken tender in the flour mixture, making sure it's well coated on all sides. Shake off any excess flour.

5. Place the coated chicken tenders on one side of the prepared baking sheet.

6. In a separate bowl, toss the sweet potato wedges with olive oil until they are evenly coated.

7. Arrange the sweet potato wedges on the other side of the baking sheet.

8. Place the baking sheet in the preheated oven and bake the chicken tenders and sweet potato wedges for about 15-20 minutes or until the chicken is cooked through and the sweet potato wedges are tender and slightly crispy.

9. Once the chicken tenders and sweet potato wedges are done, remove them from the oven.

10. Your Baked Chicken Tenders with Sweet Potato Wedges are now ready to serve!

**Inspire young chefs to appreciate the art of healthy cooking in their Baked Chicken Tenders with Sweet Potato Wedges, and to take pride in creating wholesome and balanced meals. Cooking is an opportunity to create delicious and nutritious masterpieces. Happy baking and culinary creativity!

40

Caprese Salad with Balsamic Glaze

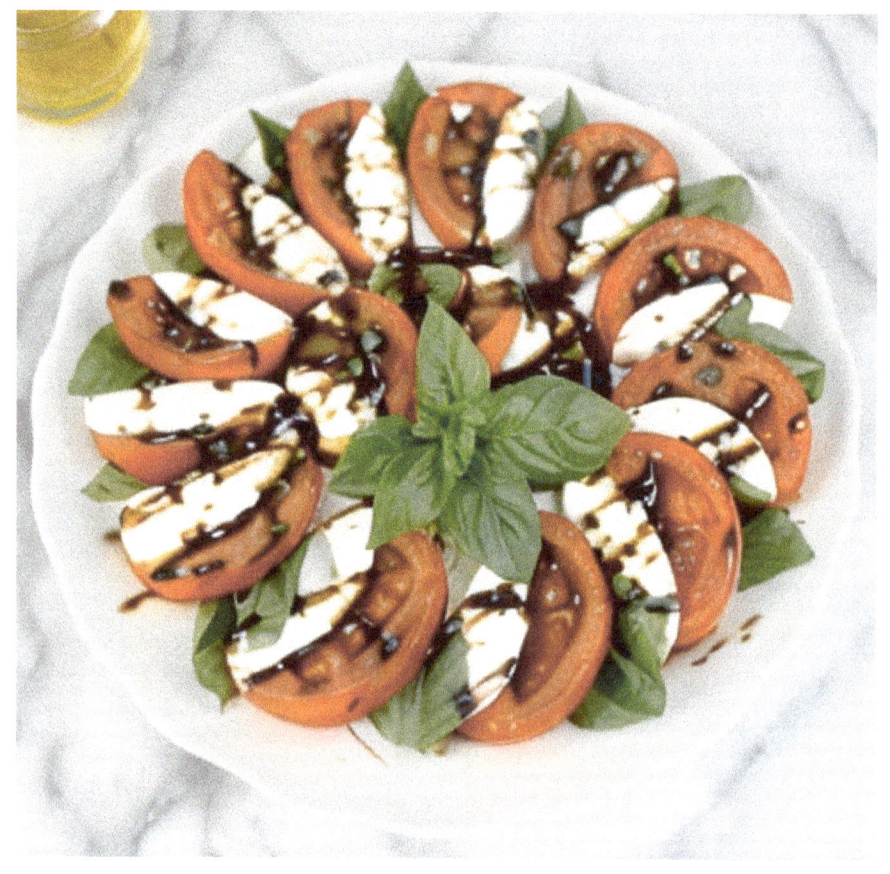

Caprese Salad with Balsamic Glaze

CAPRESE SALAD WITH BALSAMIC GLAZE

"In every Caprese Salad, you have the power to create a masterpiece with the harmony of colors and tastes. Embrace the art of simplicity, and with every bite, taste the tantalizing flavors in your culinary creation!" - Papa True Ju

In Chapter 40, we celebrate the vibrant harmony of flavors in the delectable Caprese Salad with Balsamic Glaze—a dish that perfectly encapsulates my sons' love for salads of all kinds.

One sunny afternoon, we strolled through the local farmer's market, handpicking the freshest ingredients for our salad adventure. We knew that tomatoes, mozzarella, and basil would be the stars of this delightful dish.

The sweet, juicy tomatoes were carefully sliced, revealing their vibrant red hue. As we arranged them on the platter, my sons' excitement grew, eager to taste the first bites of this mouthwatering creation.

Next came the creamy mozzarella, delicate and soft. My sons delighted in tearing it into bite-sized pieces, savoring a few morsels along the way.

For the final touch, we lovingly plucked fresh basil leaves and gently placed them atop the tomato and mozzarella, releasing their aromatic essence.

As we marveled at the beauty of our creation, my sons couldn't resist a taste. The combination of ripe tomatoes, creamy mozzarella, and aromatic basil was a burst of summer on their taste buds.

But there was more to come—a drizzle of rich, sweet balsamic glaze that added the perfect balance to this classic salad. As the glaze cascaded over the ingredients, it brought a touch of elegance and a symphony of flavors to the dish.

My sons were overjoyed with this newfound culinary delight, and they proudly declared that Caprese Salad with Balsamic Glaze would become a staple in our family's kitchen.

This salad, simple in its preparation, exemplifies the beauty of combining fresh, quality ingredients to create something truly extraordinary. As you and your young chefs prepare this vibrant Caprese Salad with Balsamic Glaze, may it transport you to warm summer days, filled with the joy of shared meals and the magic of fresh, wholesome flavors. Bon appétit!

Caprese Salad with Balsamic Glaze:

Ingredients:
- 2 large ripe tomatoes, washed and sliced
- 1 ball of fresh mozzarella cheese, sliced
- Fresh basil leaves
- Balsamic glaze
- Extra-virgin olive oil
- Salt and pepper to taste

Instructions:

1. Wash and slice the ripe tomatoes into evenly sized-slices.

2. Slice the fresh mozzarella cheese into similar-sized slices as the tomatoes.

3. Wash the fresh basil leaves and pat them dry with a paper towel.

4. On a serving platter, alternate layers of tomato slices, mozzarella slices, and fresh basil leaves to create a visually appealing pattern.

5. Drizzle extra-virgin olive oil over the salad, giving it a light and flavorful coating.

CAPRESE SALAD WITH BALSAMIC GLAZE

6. Season the Caprese Salad with a pinch of salt and pepper to enhance the flavors.

7. For an added touch of sweetness and depth of flavor, drizzle balsamic glaze over the salad. Start with a little, and you can always add more to taste.

8. Your Caprese Salad with Balsamic Glaze is now ready to enjoy!

**Inspire young chefs to appreciate the art of simplicity in their Caprese Salad with Balsamic Glaze, and to take pride in creating a masterpiece with the harmony of colors and tastes. Cooking is an opportunity to create beautiful and delicious masterpieces. Happy slicing and culinary creativity!

41

Veggie Chili with Cornbread

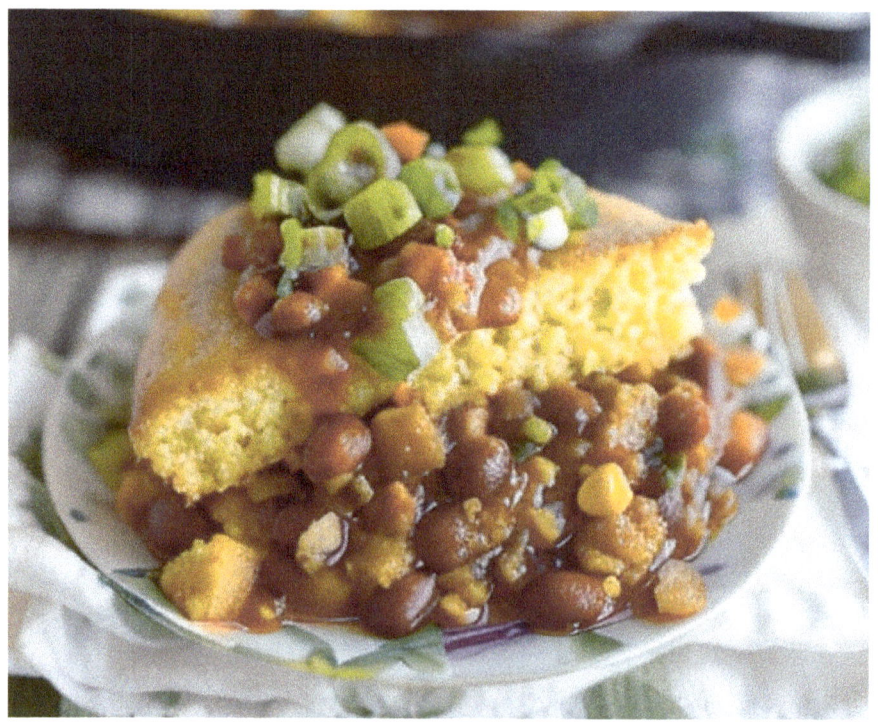

Veggie Chili with Cornbread

VEGGIE CHILI WITH CORNBREAD

"*In every veggie chili and cornbread pairing, you have the power to warm hearts with your nourishing creations. Embrace the art of comforting flavors, and be happy with your culinary creation!*" - Coach Rae

In Chapter 41, we celebrate the heartwarming and comforting flavors of Veggie Chili with Cornbread—a recipe that has become a cherished favorite on our "vegetarian night" at home.

On one chilly evening, as we gathered around the table, the aroma of simmering vegetables and spices filled the air. My sons eagerly watched as their mother prepared a steaming pot of Veggie Chili, each ingredient chosen with love and care.

The foundation of this hearty chili lies in the medley of colorful vegetables: hearty black beans, tender kidney beans, and vibrant bell peppers. As they mingled with the aromatic onions and garlic, my sons' anticipation grew.

To add depth and complexity, their mother included a blend of flavorful spices: cumin, paprika, and chili powder. The symphony of scents filled the kitchen, and my sons knew something truly special was about to be served.

As the chili simmered, we set out to prepare the perfect accompaniment: fluffy, golden cornbread. The boys loved how the cornmeal blended harmoniously with buttermilk, creating a delightful, slightly sweet contrast to the savory chili.

Finally, the moment arrived. As we spooned the Veggie Chili into bowls and placed slices of warm cornbread beside them, my sons' faces lit up with delight. Each bite was a medley of flavors—a perfect balance of wholesome vegetables, rich spices, and hearty goodness.

My sons were instantly hooked on this delicious creation, and they couldn't thank us enough for introducing them to Veggie Chili with Cornbread. From that day on, it became a beloved tradition on our "vegetarian night," where we celebrate the beauty of plant-based meals that are both nourishing and satisfying.

As you and your young chefs prepare this Veggie Chili with Cornbread, may it become a cherished part of your family gatherings, filling your home with the warmth and joy of shared meals and treasured moments. Enjoy this hearty and wholesome dish, created with love and the simple goodness of fresh, flavorful ingredients. Bon appétit!

Veggie Chili with Cornbread:

Veggie Chili Ingredients:
- 1 tablespoon olive oil
- 1 small onion, diced
- 2 cloves garlic, minced
- 1 bell pepper, diced
- 1 zucchini, diced
- 1 carrot, diced
- 1 can (15 ounces) diced tomatoes
- 1 can (15 ounces) kidney beans, drained and rinsed
- 1 can (15 ounces) black beans, drained and rinsed
- 2 tablespoons chili powder
- 1 teaspoon ground cumin
- 1/2 teaspoon paprika
- Salt and pepper to taste
- Optional toppings: shredded cheese, sliced green onions, or cilantro

Cornbread Ingredients:
- 1 cup cornmeal
- 1 cup all-purpose flour
- 1/4 cup granulated sugar

VEGGIE CHILI WITH CORNBREAD

- 1 tablespoon baking powder
- 1/2 teaspoon salt
- 1 cup milk (regular or plant-based)
- 1/4 cup unsalted butter, melted (or vegetable oil for a dairy-free option)
- 1 large egg

Instructions:

Veggie Chili:

1. In a large pot, heat the olive oil over medium heat.

2. Add the diced onion and minced garlic, and sauté until they become translucent and fragrant.

3. Stir in the diced bell pepper, zucchini, and carrot. Cook for a few minutes until the vegetables start to soften.

4. Add the diced tomatoes, kidney beans, and black beans to the pot, stirring everything together.

5. Season the chili with chili powder, ground cumin, paprika, salt, and pepper. Stir well to distribute the spices evenly.

6. Allow the chili to simmer on low heat for about 20-25 minutes, allowing the flavors to meld together.

7. While the chili is simmering, you can prepare the cornbread.

Cornbread:

1. Preheat your oven to 375°F (190°C). Grease a square baking dish (8x8 inches) with cooking spray or butter.

2. In a large mixing bowl, combine the cornmeal, all-purpose flour, sugar, baking powder, and salt.

3. In a separate bowl, whisk together the milk, melted butter (or vegetable oil), and egg.

4. Pour the wet ingredients into the dry ingredients, stirring just until combined. Be careful not to overmix.

5. Pour the cornbread batter into the greased baking dish, spreading it out evenly.

6. Bake the cornbread in the preheated oven for about 20-25 minutes or until a toothpick inserted into the center comes out clean.

7. Once the cornbread is done, remove it from the oven and let it cool slightly before serving.

Serving:

1. Ladle the Veggie Chili into bowls.

2. Cut the cornbread into squares or wedges.

3. Serve the Veggie Chili with a side of warm cornbread.

4. If desired, you can top the chili with shredded cheese, sliced green onions, or cilantro for extra flavor and color.

**Inspire young chefs to appreciate the art of comforting flavors in their Veggie Chili with Cornbread, and to take pride in warming hearts with their nourishing creations. Cooking is an opportunity to create comforting and heartwarming masterpieces. Happy simmering, baking, and culinary creativity!

42

Baked Falafel with Tahini Dressing

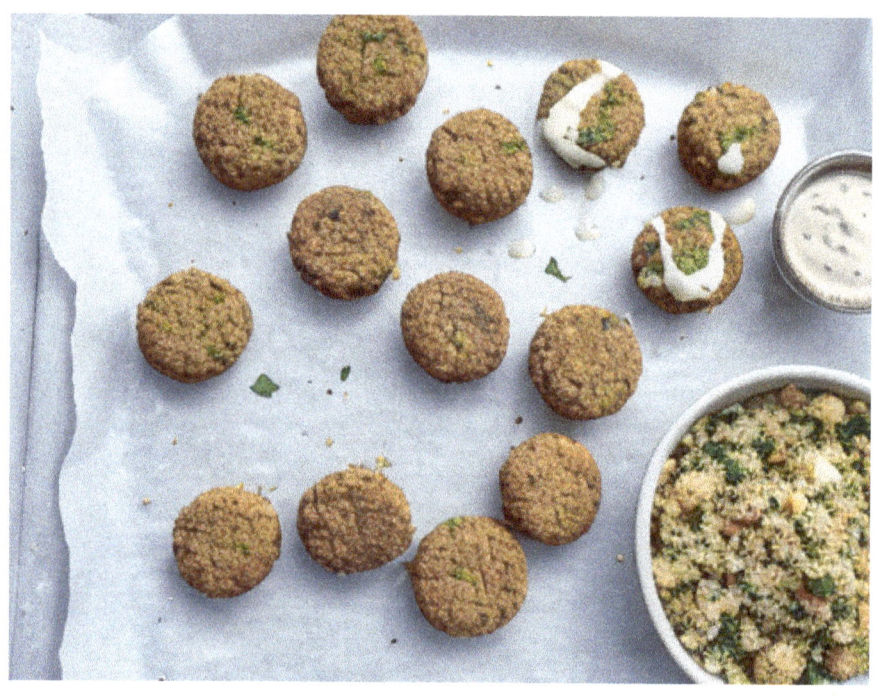

Baked Falafel with Tahini Dressing

"In every baked falafel and creamy tahini dressing, you have the power to take taste buds on an exciting journey. Embrace the art of plant-

based goodness, and enjoy eating your healthy culinary creation!" - Divine Family Unit

Chapter 42 brings an exciting twist to our culinary adventure with Baked Falafel and Tahini Dressing—a delightful dish that introduced my sons to the flavors of the Middle East.

One sunny afternoon, we decided to venture into the world of falafel—a dish that intrigued us with its rich history and exotic taste. As we gathered in the kitchen, the boys were excited to try something new, yet not too extreme for their developing palates.

Our Baked Falafel starts with a blend of hearty chickpeas and fragrant herbs, including fresh parsley and earthy cumin. These ingredients combine to create delectable falafel patties, which we bake to a perfect golden brown for a healthier twist.

The tahini dressing, made with smooth sesame paste, tangy lemon juice, and a hint of garlic, adds a creamy and nutty flavor that perfectly complements the crispy falafel.

As the boys took their first bites, their taste buds were delighted by the harmonious medley of flavors. The crunchy exterior of the falafel revealed a tender and flavorful interior, while the tahini dressing added a creamy and savory finish.

The boys couldn't get enough of this fantastic dish, and their love for trying new foods grew even stronger. Baked Falafel with Tahini Dressing became an instant favorite, a meal that allowed them to savor diverse flavors familiarly and enjoyably.

Through this experience, we discovered that introducing our children to global cuisines doesn't have to be overwhelming. Instead, it can be a fun and delicious journey of discovery, expanding their culinary horizons one bite at a time.

As you and your young chefs embark on this flavorful adventure with Baked Falafel and Tahini Dressing, may it spark a newfound appreciation for the beauty of international flavors and the joy of sharing diverse meals with loved ones. Embrace the variance and excitement that new foods bring, and savor the taste of this wholesome and delectable dish. Bon appétit!

Baked Falafel with Tahini Dressing:

Baked Falafel Ingredients:
   - 1 can (15 ounces) chickpeas, drained and rinsed
   - 1/4 cup fresh parsley leaves
   - 1/4 cup fresh cilantro leaves
   - 1 small onion, chopped
   - 3 cloves garlic
   - 1 teaspoon ground cumin
   - 1 teaspoon ground coriander
   - 1/2 teaspoon baking powder
   - 1 tablespoon lemon juice
   - 2 tablespoons all-purpose flour (or chickpea flour for a gluten-free option)
   - Salt and pepper to taste
   - 2 tablespoons olive oil

Tahini Dressing Ingredients:
   - 1/4 cup tahini
   - 2 tablespoons lemon juice
   - 2 tablespoons water
   - 1 clove garlic, minced
   - Salt to taste

Instructions:

Baked Falafel:

1. Preheat your oven to 375°F (190°C). Line a baking sheet with parchment paper or lightly grease it with cooking spray.

2. In a food processor, combine the chickpeas, fresh parsley, fresh cilantro, chopped onion, garlic, ground cumin, ground coriander, baking powder, lemon juice, all-purpose flour, salt, and pepper.

3. Pulse the mixture until it becomes a coarse texture, with the ingredients well combined. Be careful not to over-process; you want some texture in the falafel mixture.

4. Using clean hands, shape the falafel mixture into small balls or patties, about the size of a walnut.

5. Place the shaped falafel on the prepared baking sheet.

6. Drizzle olive oil over the falafel to help them bake to a crispy and golden brown.

7. Bake the falafel in the preheated oven for about 20-25 minutes, flipping them halfway through baking to ensure even browning.

Tahini Dressing:

1. In a small bowl, whisk together the tahini, lemon juice, water, minced garlic, and salt until it forms a smooth and creamy dressing. Add more water if needed to achieve your desired consistency.

Serving:

1. Serve the freshly baked falafel on a platter or in pita pockets.

2. Drizzle the tahini dressing over the falafel for a creamy and tangy flavor.

3. You can also add lettuce, tomatoes, cucumbers, or any other favorite veggies to complete the falafel wraps.

**Inspire young chefs to appreciate the art of plant-based goodness in their Baked Falafel with Tahini Dressing, and to take pride in taking taste buds on an exciting and flavorful journey. Cooking is an opportunity to create delicious and satisfying masterpieces. Happy baking, dressing, and culinary creativity!

43

Greek Salad with Olives and Feta Cheese

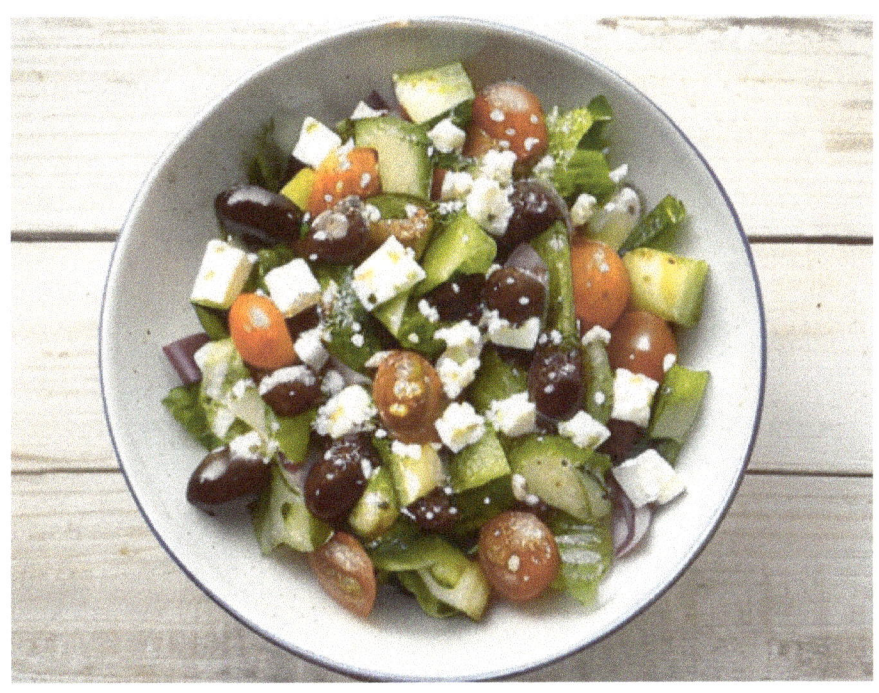

Greek Salad with Olives and Feta Cheese

"*In every Greek salad with olives and feta cheese, you have the power to savor the taste of Mediterranean delight. Embrace the art of freshness with every bite of your culinary creation!" - Coach Rae*

Chapter 43 celebrates the vibrant flavors of the Mediterranean with our Greek Salad with Olives and Feta Cheese—a delightful creation that opened the door to a world of new tastes for my adventurous sons.

One summer evening, we decided to embrace the spirit of the Mediterranean and explore the wonders of Greek cuisine. As we prepared the Greek Salad together, the boys' curiosity grew as they discovered the distinctive ingredients that make this dish so special.

Fresh, crisp cucumbers and juicy tomatoes served as the base of our salad, bringing a refreshing and wholesome touch to each bite. The boys were intrigued by the addition of tangy Kalamata olives, whose rich flavor provided a delightful contrast to the salad's crispness.

The crowning jewel of our Greek Salad was the creamy and savory feta cheese, which my sons adored. Its unique taste added a burst of indulgence to the vibrant mix of ingredients, creating a harmonious and unforgettable flavor profile.

Drizzled with a light and zesty dressing made of olive oil, lemon juice, and fragrant oregano, the salad came together in a symphony of tastes that left the boys wanting more.

As they savored their first bites, their faces lit up with joy and excitement, appreciating the deliciousness of this Mediterranean delight. Greek Salad with Olives and Feta Cheese quickly became a staple in our kitchen, a refreshing and nutritious option that the boys were always eager to prepare and enjoy.

This dish taught us that trying new foods can be an adventure filled with delightful surprises and endless possibilities. Each ingredient brings its unique character to the table, forming a tapestry of flavors that dance on the taste buds.

As you embark on your own Greek Salad journey, may it inspire a love for exploring the rich and diverse world of cuisines. Embrace the delightful combination of ingredients, and savor the joy of sharing this wholesome and enticing salad with your loved ones. Bon appétit!

Greek Salad with Olives and Feta Cheese:

Ingredients:
- 2 large cucumbers, washed and diced
- 4 large ripe tomatoes, washed and diced
- 1 small red onion, thinly sliced
- 1 cup Kalamata olives, pitted
- 1/2 cup crumbled feta cheese
- Fresh parsley leaves for garnish (optional)

For the Dressing:
- 1/4 cup extra-virgin olive oil
- 2 tablespoons red wine vinegar
- 1 teaspoon dried oregano
- Salt and pepper to taste

Instructions:

1. In a large mixing bowl, combine the diced cucumbers, diced tomatoes, and thinly sliced red onion.

2. Add the pitted Kalamata olives to the bowl.

3. In a small bowl, whisk together the extra-virgin olive oil, red wine vinegar, dried oregano, salt, and pepper to make the dressing.

4. Pour the dressing over the salad ingredients in the large mixing bowl.

5. Gently toss the salad to ensure all the ingredients are evenly coated with the dressing.

6. Sprinkle the crumbled feta cheese over the salad.

7. If desired, garnish with fresh parsley leaves for an extra touch of color and flavor.

8. Your Greek Salad with Olives and Feta Cheese is now ready to serve!

**Inspire young chefs to appreciate the art of freshness in their Greek Salad with Olives and Feta Cheese, and to take pride in savoring the taste of Mediterranean delight. Cooking is an opportunity to create refreshing and delightful masterpieces. Happy salad-making and culinary creativity!

44

Cauliflower Crust Pizza with Veggie Toppings

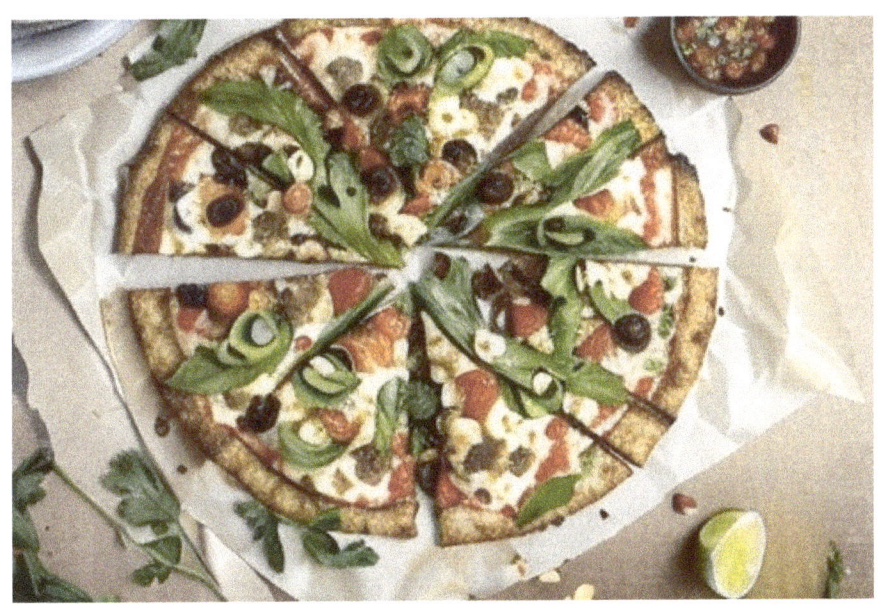

Cauliflower Crust Pizza with Veggie Toppings

"*In every cauliflower crust pizza with veggie toppings, you have the power to turn veggies into a delightful canvas of flavors. Embrace the*

***art of creativity, and add a cool twist to your culinary creation!"* -
Papa True Ju***

In Chapter 44, we embark on a pizza adventure like no other, as we introduce you to our Cauliflower Crust Pizza with Veggie Toppings—a delightful twist on a beloved classic that captured the hearts of my pizza-loving sons.

One Friday night, we decided to have a homemade pizza party, and I suggested we try something new. The boys were thrilled at the idea of making their pizza, but they were in for a delightful surprise when they learned about our innovative crust.

As we gathered in the kitchen, the boys eagerly helped prepare the cauliflower crust—a brilliant and wholesome alternative to traditional pizza dough. Grating fresh cauliflower and mixing it with egg, cheese, and a touch of savory herbs created a magical foundation for our pizza.

Once baked to a golden crisp, we topped our cauliflower crust with an array of colorful and nutritious veggies. Sweet bell peppers, juicy cherry tomatoes, earthy mushrooms, and vibrant spinach danced across the pizza, promising a burst of flavors and nutrients.

The boys were excited to embrace this unique texture and taste. With every bite, they marveled at the light and crispy crust that perfectly complemented the medley of fresh vegetables. They realized that a cauliflower crust pizza could be just as delicious and satisfying as the traditional one they had known.

As the boys enjoyed their Cauliflower Crust Pizza with Veggie Toppings, they felt a sense of pride in discovering a healthier yet mouthwatering twist on their favorite meal. This experience encouraged them to explore new possibilities and flavors, all while knowing that nutritious choices can be just as delightful.

CAULIFLOWER CRUST PIZZA WITH VEGGIE TOPPINGS

In this chapter, we celebrate the joy of creativity in the kitchen and the magic that happens when you take a beloved dish and reimagine it with wholesome ingredients. Cauliflower Crust Pizza with Veggie Toppings has become a cherished recipe in our home, reminding us that sometimes the most wonderful surprises can be found in the simplest of ingredients.

As you delve into the world of Cauliflower Crust Pizza, may it inspire your culinary adventures, encouraging you and your little chefs to savor every moment of discovery and share the goodness of this wholesome and scrumptious pizza with your family and friends. Buon appetito!

Cauliflower Crust Pizza with Veggie Toppings:

Cauliflower Crust Ingredients:
- 1 medium head of cauliflower, washed and grated (or riced)
- 1 large egg, lightly beaten
- 1 cup shredded mozzarella cheese
- 1 teaspoon dried oregano
- 1/2 teaspoon garlic powder
- Salt and pepper to taste

Pizza Toppings:
- 1/2 cup pizza sauce (store-bought or homemade)
- 1 cup shredded mozzarella cheese
- Assorted vegetable toppings of your choice: sliced bell peppers, sliced tomatoes, sliced onions, sliced mushrooms, sliced black olives, etc.

Instructions:

Cauliflower Crust:

1. Preheat your oven to 425°F (220°C). Line a baking sheet with parchment paper or lightly grease it with cooking spray.

2. Grate the medium head of cauliflower using a box grater or a food processor with a grating attachment. Alternatively, you can use pre-riced cauliflower.

3. In a microwave-safe bowl, microwave the grated cauliflower for 4-5 minutes on high power. Let it cool slightly before handling.

4. Place the microwaved cauliflower in a clean kitchen towel or cheesecloth. Squeeze out as much excess moisture as possible. This step is essential to achieve a crispy cauliflower crust.

5. In a mixing bowl, combine the squeezed cauliflower, lightly beaten egg, shredded mozzarella cheese, dried oregano, garlic powder, salt, and pepper.

6. Mix all the ingredients until well combined and the mixture resembles a dough-like consistency.

7. Transfer the cauliflower crust mixture to the prepared baking sheet.

8. Spread and shape the mixture into a thin, round crust or any desired shape using your hands. Aim for about 1/4-inch thickness.

9. Bake the cauliflower crust in the preheated oven for about 15-20 minutes or until it becomes golden brown and holds its shape.

Assembling and Toppings:

1. Once the cauliflower crust is baked, remove it from the oven.

2. Spread the pizza sauce evenly over the crust.

3. Sprinkle shredded mozzarella cheese on top of the sauce.

CAULIFLOWER CRUST PIZZA WITH VEGGIE TOPPINGS

4. Add your favorite vegetable toppings on the cheese layer, creating a colorful and tasty pizza.

5. Return the topped pizza to the oven and bake for an additional 10-15 minutes or until the cheese is melted, and the toppings are cooked to your liking.

6. Once the pizza is done, remove it from the oven and let it cool slightly before slicing and serving.

**Inspire young chefs to appreciate the art of creativity in their Cauliflower Crust Pizza with Veggie Toppings, and to take pride in turning veggies into a delightful canvas of flavors. Cooking is an opportunity to create delicious and artistic masterpieces. Happy pizza-making and culinary creativity!

45

Chicken and Vegetable Kebabs

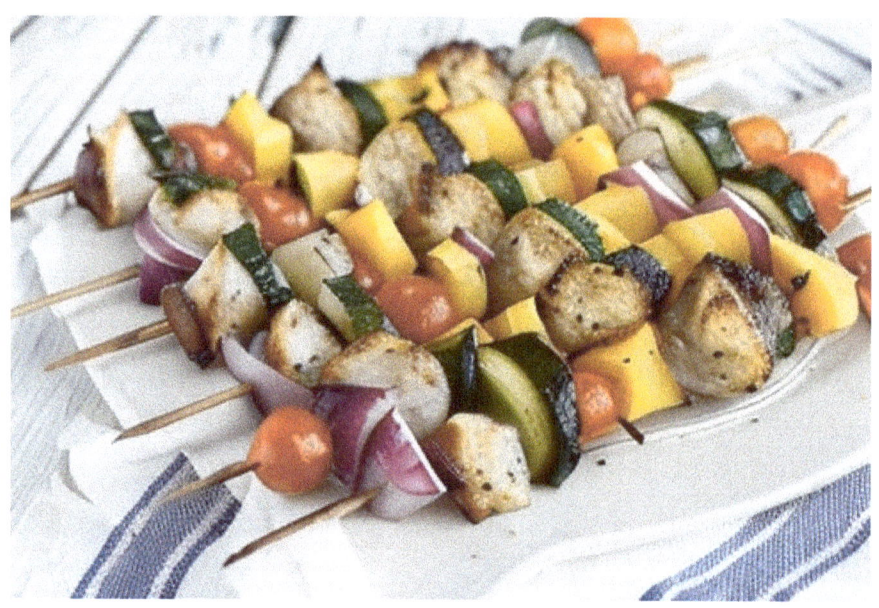

Chicken and Vegetable Kebabs

"In every chicken and vegetable kebab, you have the power to combine flavors and create a symphony of tastes. Embrace the art of grilling, and enjoy the vibrancy of your culinary creation!" - *Coach Rae*

CHICKEN AND VEGETABLE KEBABS

In Chapter 45, we embark on a delightful culinary journey with our Chicken and Vegetable Kebabs—a dish that holds a special place in the hearts of my sons since the very first time they tasted its flavorful goodness.

One sunny afternoon, we decided to fire up the grill and experiment with some new kebab recipes. As we prepared the ingredients, the boys were eager to help skewer the succulent pieces of tender chicken, bell peppers, zucchini, and juicy cherry tomatoes onto the wooden sticks.

The secret to the mouthwatering flavor of these kebabs lies in the marinade we lovingly prepared. A blend of zesty lemon juice, fragrant garlic, earthy herbs, and a hint of honey harmoniously infused the chicken and vegetables, creating a symphony of tastes that would delight the taste buds.

As the kebabs sizzled on the grill, the aroma filled the air, heightening the anticipation. The boys couldn't wait to take their first bite of the colorful and enticing skewers.

When the Chicken and Vegetable Kebabs were finally ready, we gathered around the table, and the boys dove into this culinary creation with enthusiasm. Their eyes lit up as they savored the burst of flavors—tender, juicy chicken perfectly complemented by the charred sweetness of the bell peppers, the crispness of zucchini, and the burst of tangy tomatoes.

With each mouthful, the boys appreciated how the simple combination of fresh ingredients and a touch of grilling magic could create such a delightful and satisfying meal. Chicken and Vegetable Kebabs quickly became a go-to favorite, not only for its delectable taste but also for the wonderful memories created around the grill.

In Chapter 45, we celebrate the joy of cooking together, the thrill of trying something new, and the beauty of sharing a delicious meal with loved ones. The Chicken and Vegetable Kebabs symbolize the spirit of adventure and the warmth of family gatherings, reminding us that the most cherished recipes are the ones made with love and shared with those who matter the most.

As you prepare your Chicken and Vegetable Kebabs, may the sizzle of the grill and the laughter of your loved ones fill your hearts with joy and your kitchen with the aroma of togetherness. Enjoy the delightful flavors and the happiness that comes with every bite of these tasty and wholesome kebabs. Bon appétit!

Chicken and Vegetable Kebabs:

Ingredients:
 - 1 pound boneless, skinless chicken breast, cut into bite-sized pieces
 - Assorted vegetables of your choice, cut into bite-sized pieces (e.g., bell peppers, onions, cherry tomatoes, zucchini, mushrooms)
 - Olive oil for brushing
 - Salt and pepper to taste
 - Wooden or metal skewers

Instructions:

1. If using wooden skewers, soak them in water for about 30 minutes before assembling the kebabs. This prevents them from burning while grilling.

2. Preheat your grill or grill pan over medium-high heat.

3. Assemble the kebabs by threading the bite-sized chicken pieces and assorted vegetables onto the skewers in any order you prefer.

4. Brush the assembled kebabs with olive oil to prevent sticking and add a touch of flavor.

5. Season the kebabs with salt and pepper to taste, enhancing the flavors.

6. Place the kebabs on the preheated grill or grill pan and cook for about 8-10 minutes, turning occasionally, until the chicken is cooked through and the vegetables are tender and slightly charred.

7. Once the kebabs are cooked, remove them from the grill and let them rest for a few minutes.

8. Serve the Chicken and Vegetable Kebabs on a platter and enjoy!

**Inspire young chefs to appreciate the art of grilling in their Chicken and Vegetable Kebabs, and to take pride in combining flavors to create a symphony of tastes. Cooking is an opportunity to create delicious and harmonious masterpieces. Happy grilling and culinary creativity!

46

Veggie-Loaded Macaroni and Cheese

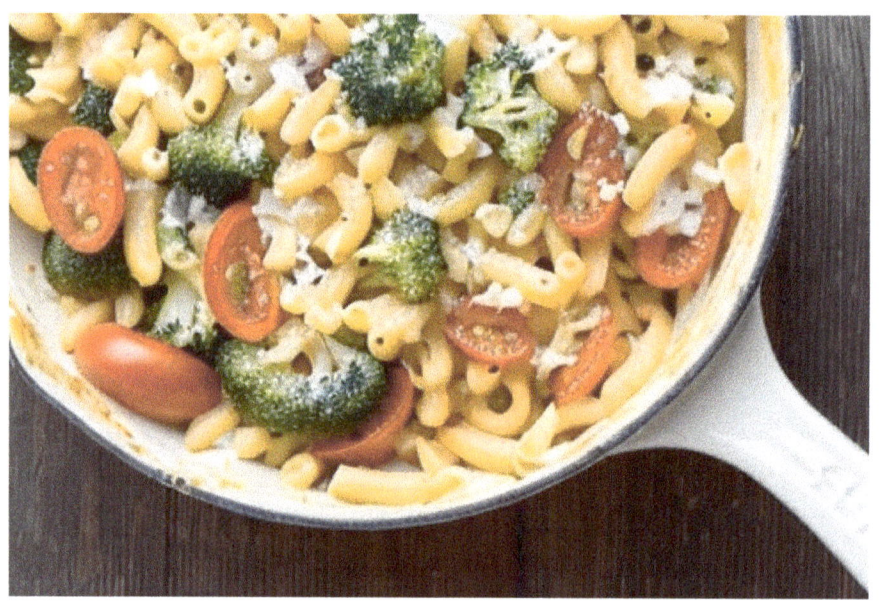

Veggie-Loaded Macaroni and Cheese

"*In every veggie-loaded macaroni and cheese, you have the power to turn comfort food into a colorful and nutritious delight. Embrace the art of balance within your culinary creation!*"
- *Divine Family Unit*

VEGGIE-LOADED MACARONI AND CHEESE

Chapter 46 takes us on a scrumptious adventure as we delve into the world of Veggie-Loaded Macaroni and Cheese—a delightful twist on a beloved classic that never fails to excite my sons.

One evening, while enjoying a cozy family dinner, my sons mentioned how much they loved macaroni and cheese. As a parent who values a balanced meal, I saw the opportunity to sneak in some nutritious goodness while preserving the creamy, cheesy comfort they adore.

The key to this delectable dish lies in the selection of vibrant vegetables. As we prepare the macaroni, we gently stir in a medley of colorful veggies, such as crisp broccoli florets, sweet corn kernels, and tender baby spinach. Each veggie adds its unique flavor and texture, turning this humble mac and cheese into a nutrient-packed delight.

As the cheesy aroma fills the kitchen, my boy's excitement builds, knowing that their favorite dish is getting an extra boost of goodness from the veggies. It's a wonderful sight to see them eagerly anticipate every bite, discovering a new taste experience with each forkful.

When the Veggie-Loaded Macaroni and Cheese is finally ready, we gather around the table, and my sons can hardly contain their enthusiasm. The velvety, cheese-coated pasta with pops of vibrant veggies creates a harmony of flavors that make this dish truly special.

With each spoonful, my sons appreciate how simple swaps can transform classic comfort food into a wholesome and satisfying meal. They also take pride in the fact that they are eating a meal that not only tastes good but also makes them feel good inside.

Chapter 46 celebrates the joy of creativity in the kitchen and the beauty of turning an iconic meal into something new and exciting. Veggie-Loaded Macaroni and Cheese showcases the magic of blending familiar comfort with wholesome goodness, reminding us that sometimes the best meals are the ones that combine the familiar and the adventurous.

As you prepare your Veggie-Loaded Macaroni and Cheese, may the smiles of your loved ones and the appreciation for a balanced and flavorful dish warm your heart. Enjoy the comfort of classic mac and cheese, knowing that it's now infused with the goodness of colorful vegetables, making it a true family favorite. Bon appétit!

Veggie-Loaded Macaroni and Cheese:

Ingredients:
 - 8 ounces of elbow macaroni or your favorite pasta
 - 2 cups mixed vegetables (e.g., broccoli florets, diced bell peppers, peas, carrots)
 - 2 tablespoons unsalted butter
 - 2 tablespoons all-purpose flour
 - 2 cups milk
 - 2 cups shredded cheddar cheese
 - Salt and pepper to taste
 - Optional: 1/4 cup grated Parmesan cheese for added flavor

Instructions:

1. Cook the elbow macaroni or your favorite pasta according to the package instructions in a large pot of salted boiling water until al dente. Drain the pasta and set it aside.

2. While the pasta is cooking, prepare the mixed vegetables by steaming or boiling them until tender. Drain and set them aside.

3. In the same pot used for cooking the pasta, melt the unsalted butter over medium heat.

VEGGIE-LOADED MACARONI AND CHEESE

4. Stir in the all-purpose flour and cook for about 1-2 minutes, stirring constantly, to form a roux.

5. Gradually add the milk to the roux, stirring continuously to avoid lumps.

6. Cook the sauce over medium heat until it thickens and begins to bubble.

7. Reduce the heat to low, and add the shredded cheddar cheese to the sauce. Stir until the cheese is fully melted and the sauce becomes smooth and creamy.

8. Season the cheese sauce with salt and pepper to taste. You can also add the grated Parmesan cheese at this point for extra flavor.

9. Add the cooked pasta and mixed vegetables to the cheese sauce, stirring gently to coat everything evenly.

10. Your Veggie-Loaded Macaroni and Cheese is now ready to serve!

**Inspire young chefs to appreciate the art of balance in their Veggie-Loaded Macaroni and Cheese, and to take pride in turning comfort food into a colorful and nutritious delight. Cooking is an opportunity to create delicious and well-rounded masterpieces. Happy cooking and culinary creativity!

47

Banana and Almond Butter Smoothie

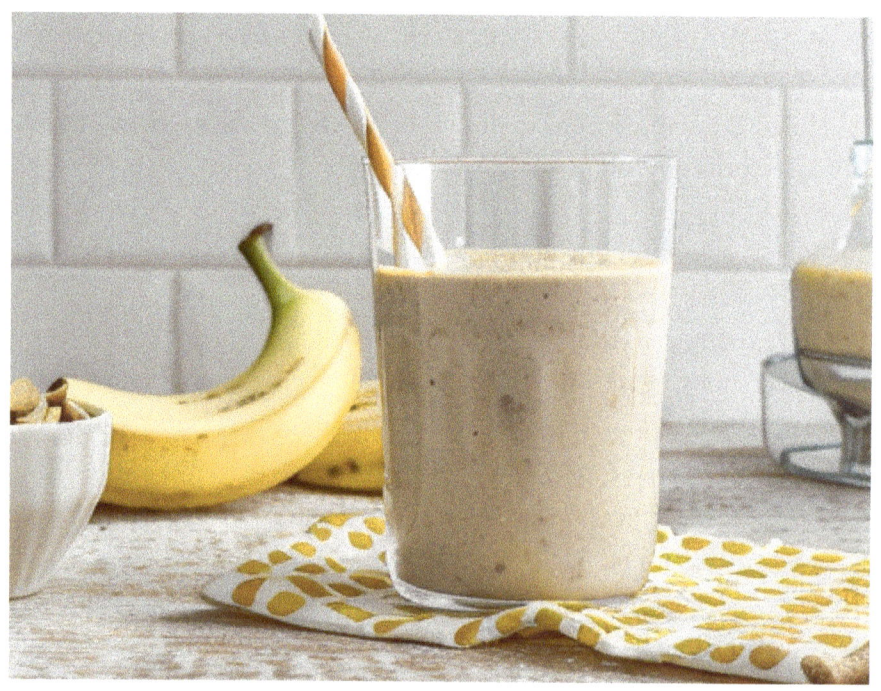

Banana and Almond Butter Smoothie

"*In every banana and almond butter smoothie, you have the power to blend health and happiness in a single sip. Embrace the art of*

BANANA AND ALMOND BUTTER SMOOTHIE

nourishment, and with every sip, know you did your best!" - Coach Rae

Chapter 47 takes us on a delightful journey into the world of the Banana and Almond Butter Smoothie—a refreshing and energizing treat that has quickly become a favorite for my sons.

One sunny afternoon, my sons watched in awe as I prepared this creamy and wholesome smoothie for myself. Intrigued by the combination of flavors, they couldn't resist asking for a taste. As they sipped the frosty goodness, their faces lit up with sheer delight.

The magic of this smoothie lies in the simplicity of its ingredients. Sweet, ripe bananas bring a natural creaminess and a burst of energy to the blend. Paired with smooth, nutty almond butter, the flavor combination is simply divine.

The addition of almond milk lends a velvety texture and a touch of nutty flavor, perfectly complementing the bananas and almond butter. A drizzle of honey adds a gentle sweetness, making this smoothie a well-rounded treat that satisfies the taste buds and nourishes the body.

As my sons enjoyed their Banana and Almond Butter Smoothie, they couldn't help but feel the energy flowing through them. They loved how the smoothie provided a quick pick-me-up, making it an ideal choice before heading out to play or during a busy afternoon of activities.

From that moment on, this smoothie has been a staple in our home, bringing joy and refreshment with every sip. My sons eagerly prepare it for themselves, relishing the feeling of independence and accomplishment as they create a delicious and nutritious treat.

Chapter 47 celebrates the joy of discovering new flavors and embracing wholesome ingredients in a simple yet delightful way. The Banana and Almond Butter Smoothie captures the essence of a nourishing and satisfying meal that keeps my sons energized and excited throughout their day.

As you blend your Banana and Almond Butter Smoothie, may the smiles on your children's faces and the sense of vitality it brings remind you of the simple joys found in nourishing and delicious meals. Savor the delightful taste of this smoothie and relish the happiness it brings. Enjoy this delightful treat that has quickly become a cherished part of our family's daily routine. Cheers to good health and happy moments together!

Banana and Almond Butter Smoothie:

Ingredients:
- 2 ripe bananas, peeled and sliced
- 2 tablespoons almond butter
- 1 cup milk (dairy or plant-based)
- 1 tablespoon honey or maple syrup (optional for added sweetness)
- Ice cubes (optional for a colder smoothie)

Instructions:

1. In a blender, combine the sliced ripe bananas, almond butter, and milk.

2. If desired, add honey or maple syrup for added sweetness.

3. If you prefer a colder smoothie, you can also add a few ice cubes to the blender.

4. Blend all the ingredients until smooth and creamy.

5. If the smoothie is too thick, you can add more milk to achieve your desired consistency.

BANANA AND ALMOND BUTTER SMOOTHIE

6. Pour the Banana and Almond Butter Smoothie into a glass.

7. Optionally, you can garnish with banana slices or a drizzle of almond butter on top.

8. Your Banana and Almond Butter Smoothie is now ready to enjoy!

**Inspire young chefs to appreciate the art of nourishment in their Banana and Almond Butter Smoothie, and to take pride in blending health and happiness in a single sip. Cooking is an opportunity to create delicious and wholesome masterpieces. Happy blending and culinary creativity!

48

Veggie and Cheese Stuffed Mushrooms

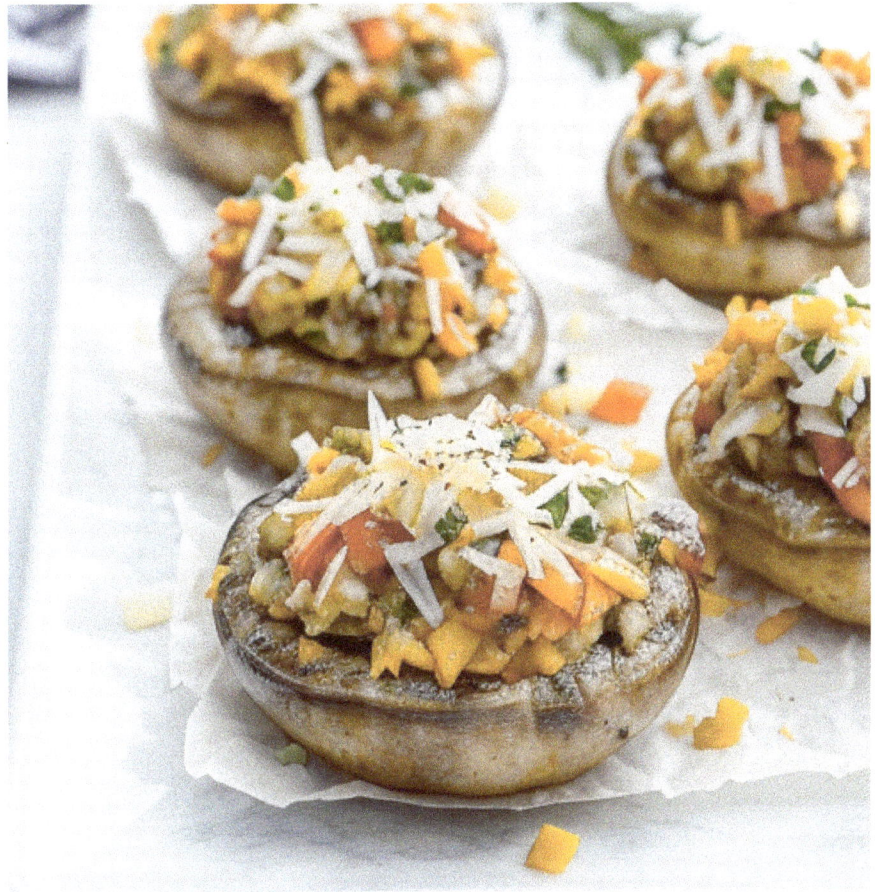

Veggie and Cheese Stuffed Mushrooms

"*In every veggie and cheese stuffed mushroom, you have the power to turn simple fungi into a delectable treasure. Embrace the art of creativity, and cook a truly unique meal!*"
- Papa True Ju

In Chapter 48, we embark on a delightful culinary adventure with Veggie and Cheese Stuffed Mushrooms—a dish that has won the hearts of my sons with its delicious blend of flavors and textures.

One cozy evening, as we were brainstorming new meal ideas, my sons stumbled upon a recipe for stuffed mushrooms in a magazine. They were intrigued by the concept of turning humble mushrooms into bite-sized vessels filled with delectable goodness.

As we prepared the dish together, my sons had a blast hollowing out the mushrooms and carefully stuffing them with a colorful medley of fresh veggies. Each mushroom became a tiny canvas for their culinary creativity, and they took pride in their artful presentation.

To enhance the flavors, we chose a combination of vibrant bell peppers, tender spinach, and zesty onions as the stuffing. The vegetables provided a burst of colors and added a delightful crunch, making each bite a tantalizing experience.

Of course, a dish wouldn't be complete without the magic of cheese! We opted for a blend of creamy feta and savory parmesan, creating a melty and cheesy filling that elevated the mushrooms to new heights of deliciousness.

Baked to perfection, the mushrooms emerged from the oven with a tantalizing aroma that filled our home with warmth and anticipation. As my sons eagerly took their first bite, their faces lit up with joy. The Veggie and Cheese Stuffed Mushrooms had exceeded their expectations, leaving them yearning for more.

From that day forward, this dish has become a go-to appetizer for family gatherings and special occasions. My sons cherish the memories of preparing and savoring these mouthwatering stuffed mushrooms together.

Chapter 48 celebrates the art of turning simple ingredients into delightful masterpieces. The Veggie and Cheese Stuffed Mushrooms are a testament to the joy of exploring new flavors and enjoying the process of cooking together.

VEGGIE AND CHEESE STUFFED MUSHROOMS

As you embark on this culinary adventure, may the spirit of creativity and togetherness infuse your kitchen with love and excitement. Savor each delicious bite of these stuffed mushrooms and relish the joy they bring to your family. Enjoy the wonder of cooking and sharing special moments with your loved ones. Bon appétit!

Veggie and Cheese Stuffed Mushrooms:

Ingredients:
- 16 large button or cremini mushrooms, cleaned and stems removed
- 1 tablespoon olive oil
- 1 small onion, finely chopped
- 1 small bell pepper, finely chopped
- 1 cup fresh spinach, chopped
- 1/2 cup shredded cheddar cheese or your favorite cheese
- Salt and pepper to taste
- Optional: 1/4 cup grated Parmesan cheese for added flavor

Instructions:

1. Preheat your oven to 375°F (190°C). Line a baking sheet with parchment paper.

2. Clean the mushrooms by gently wiping them with a damp paper towel. Remove the stems from the mushrooms and set them aside.

3. Finely chop the mushroom stems, onion, and bell pepper.

4. In a skillet, heat the olive oil over medium heat.

5. Add the chopped mushroom stems, onion, and bell pepper to the skillet. Sauté for 3-4 minutes or until the vegetables are softened.

6. Stir in the chopped fresh spinach and cook for an additional 1-2 minutes until the spinach wilts.

7. Remove the skillet from heat, and stir in the shredded cheddar cheese. Season the mixture with salt and pepper to taste. If desired, you can also add the grated Parmesan cheese at this point for extra flavor.

8. Stuff each mushroom cap with the veggie and cheese mixture, pressing it gently to fill the cavity.

9. Place the stuffed mushrooms on the prepared baking sheet.

10. Bake the stuffed mushrooms in the preheated oven for 15-20 minutes or until the mushrooms are tender and the cheese is melted and bubbly.

11. Once the mushrooms are done, remove them from the oven and let them cool slightly before serving.

**Inspire young chefs to appreciate the art of creativity in their Veggie and Cheese Stuffed Mushrooms, and to take pride in turning simple fungi into a delectable treasure. Cooking is an opportunity to create delicious and savory masterpieces. Happy cooking and culinary creativity!

49

Black Bean and Corn Salad

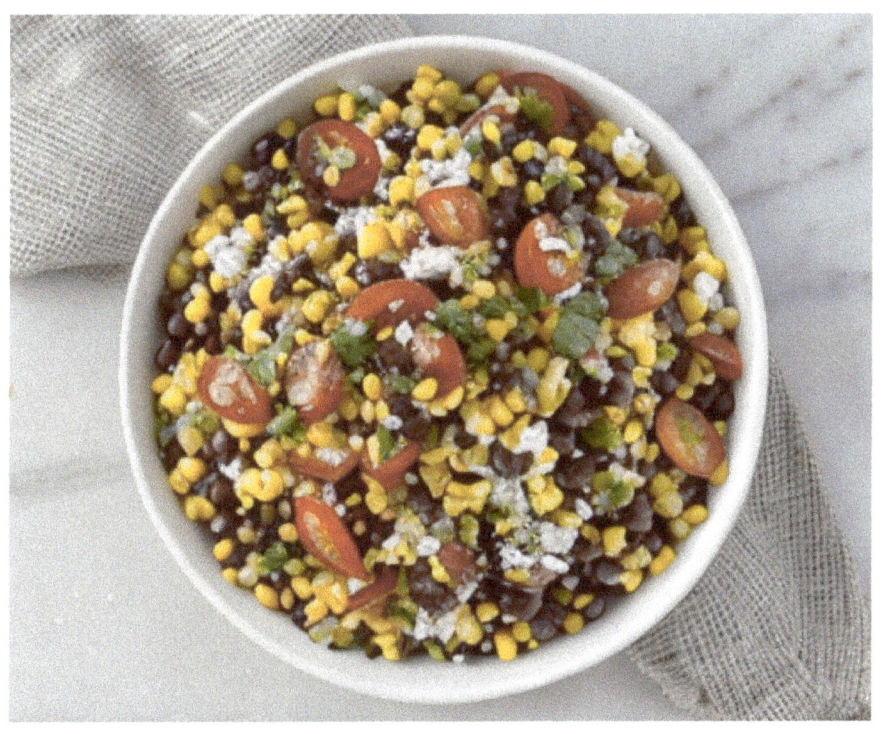

Black Bean and Corn Salad

"In every black bean and corn salad, you have the power to blend colors and flavors into a vibrant medley. Embrace the art of balance, and vibe with every bite of your culinary creation!" - Coach Rae

In Chapter 49, we embark on a flavorful journey with Black Bean and Corn Salad—a vibrant dish that holds a special place in my sons' hearts, evoking fond memories of their favorite burritos.

One sunny summer afternoon, we decided to whip up a refreshing salad to beat the heat. My sons were eager to experiment with new ingredients and create a dish reminiscent of their beloved burrito fillings.

The star ingredients in this delightful salad are hearty black beans and sweet corn, chosen for their delightful texture and nutritional benefits. These wholesome legumes bring a satisfying heartiness to the salad, perfectly mirroring the essence of a burrito.

To add a burst of color and freshness, we included juicy cherry tomatoes and crisp bell peppers. The vibrant hues not only make the salad visually appealing but also add a delightful crunch to each bite.

For a burst of tangy flavor, we dressed the salad with a zesty lime and cilantro dressing. The tanginess of the lime perfectly complements the natural sweetness of the corn and tomatoes, while the fresh cilantro adds a burst of herbaceous goodness.

As my sons took their first bite of this Black Bean and Corn Salad, they were delighted to find that it truly captured the essence of their favorite burritos. They couldn't help but reminisce about the warm tortillas, savory fillings, and the joy of building their custom burritos.

From that day on, Black Bean and Corn Salad has become a cherished go-to meal in our home. Whether it's a quick lunch, a side dish at dinner, or a delightful picnic addition, this salad never fails to bring a smile to my sons' faces.

Chapter 49 celebrates the beauty of recreating cherished flavors in a fresh and wholesome way. The Black Bean and Corn Salad embodies the spirit of creativity and nostalgia, reminding us that some of the best meals are simple, wholesome, and made with love.

As you savor this delightful salad, may it transport you to joyful memories and create new moments of togetherness with your loved ones. Enjoy the burst of flavors, the textures that dance on your palate, and the joy of sharing a meal made with love. Bon appétit!

Black Bean and Corn Salad:

Ingredients:
- 1 can (15 ounces) black beans, drained and rinsed
- 1 cup frozen corn, thawed (or canned corn, drained)
- 1 small red bell pepper, diced
- 1/4 cup finely chopped red onion
- 1/4 cup chopped fresh cilantro
- 2 tablespoons lime juice
- 2 tablespoons olive oil
- 1 teaspoon ground cumin
- Salt and pepper to taste

Instructions:

1. In a large mixing bowl, combine the black beans, thawed corn, diced red bell pepper, finely chopped red onion, and chopped fresh cilantro.

2. In a small bowl, whisk together the lime juice, olive oil, ground cumin, salt, and pepper to create the dressing.

3. Pour the dressing over the black bean and corn mixture.

4. Gently toss all the ingredients until well combined and coated with the dressing.

5. Taste and adjust the seasonings, adding more salt and pepper if desired.

6. Cover the bowl with plastic wrap or transfer the salad to an airtight container.

7. Refrigerate the Black Bean and Corn Salad for at least 30 minutes to let the flavors meld together.

8. Serve the chilled salad as a refreshing side dish or as a topping for tacos, nachos, or grilled chicken.

**Inspire young chefs to appreciate the art of balance in their Black Bean and Corn Salad, and to take pride in blending colors and flavors into a vibrant medley. Cooking is an opportunity to create delicious and well-rounded masterpieces. Happy cooking and culinary creativity!

50

Turkey and Avocado Lettuce Wraps

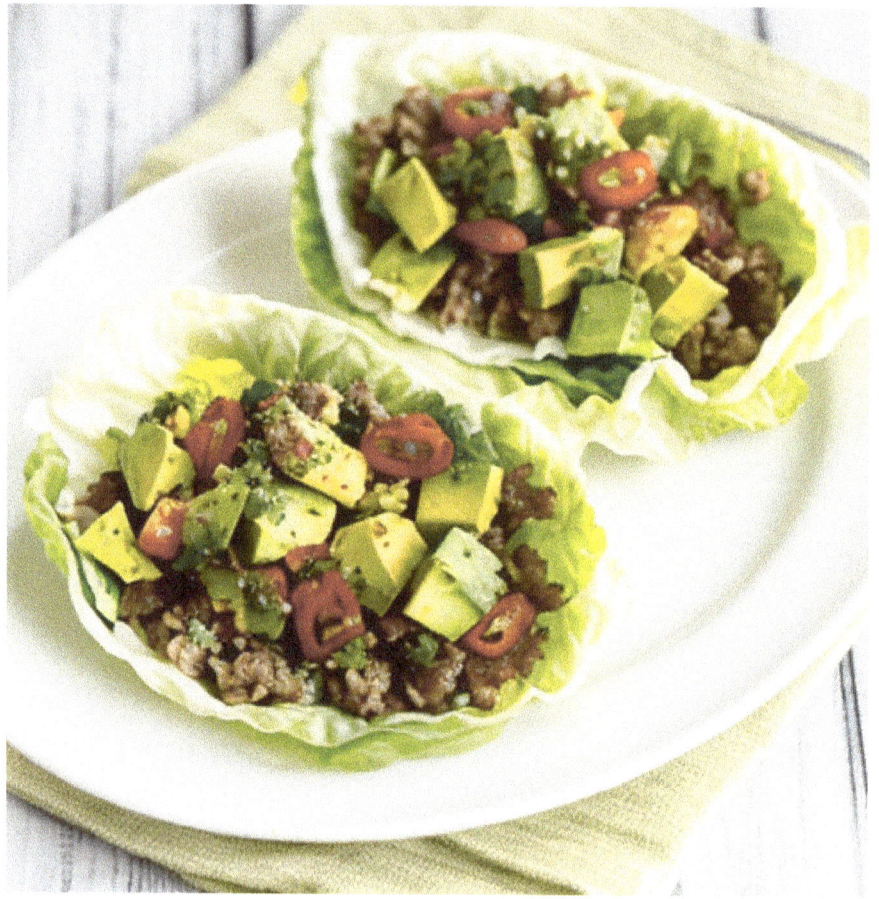

Turkey and Avocado Lettuce Wraps

"*In every turkey and avocado lettuce wrap, you have the power to create a delightful, balanced dance of flavors. Embrace the art of healthy indulgence, and do a happy dance after successfully preparing your culinary creation!*" - *Papa True Ju*

In the final chapter of our cookbook, we celebrate the joy of simplicity with Turkey and Avocado Lettuce Wraps—a delightful meal that has won my sons' hearts with its perfect harmony of flavors and ease of preparation.

One busy evening, as we were brainstorming new meal ideas, my sons

TURKEY AND AVOCADO LETTUCE WRAPS

expressed their love for simple yet flavorful combinations. They appreciated how the right ingredients could create a symphony of taste, and thus, the idea of Turkey and Avocado Lettuce Wraps was born.

At the heart of this dish is lean, tender turkey breast—carefully chosen for its wholesome protein content and ability to absorb flavors. We wanted to create a balanced, nutritious meal that would leave us feeling satisfied and energized.

For a creamy and velvety twist, we added creamy avocado slices—a superfood brimming with healthy fats and a delightful buttery taste. The avocado's rich texture perfectly complements the lean turkey, creating a luscious filling for the lettuce wraps.

To add a refreshing and crisp element, we used fresh lettuce leaves as the wraps. The crispiness of the lettuce adds a delightful contrast to the tender turkey and creamy avocado, while also providing a healthy and low-carb alternative to traditional tortillas.

A sprinkle of zesty lime juice ties all the ingredients together, infusing the wraps with a bright and tangy note. The lime's zing perfectly enhances the flavors of the turkey and avocado, turning each bite into a delicious revelation.

As my sons took their first bite of these Turkey and Avocado Lettuce Wraps, their faces lit up with delight. They were amazed at how such simple ingredients could come together to create a mouthwatering dish that they instantly fell in love with.

Chapter 50 pays tribute to the art of simplicity and the joy of discovering how a few thoughtfully chosen ingredients can bring immense pleasure to our taste buds. The Turkey and Avocado Lettuce Wraps embody the spirit of balance, nutrition, and the beauty of uncomplicated cooking.

As you savor these wraps, may you be reminded of the wonder of simplicity and the pleasure of savoring every delicious bite. Enjoy the perfect union of turkey, avocado, and lettuce—a symphony of flavors that dances on your palate and leaves you with a contented heart. Bon appétit!

Turkey and Avocado Lettuce Wraps:

Ingredients:
- 1 pound ground turkey
- 1 tablespoon olive oil
- 1 teaspoon garlic powder
- 1 teaspoon ground cumin
- 1 teaspoon paprika
- Salt and pepper to taste
- 1 large avocado, sliced
- 1 cup cherry tomatoes, halved
- 1/4 cup diced red onion
- 1/4 cup chopped fresh cilantro
- Juice of 1 lime
- Large lettuce leaves (e.g., iceberg, romaine) for wrapping

Instructions:

1. In a large skillet, heat the olive oil over medium heat.

2. Add the ground turkey to the skillet and cook until it is no longer pink, breaking it into small pieces with a spatula as it cooks.

3. Season the turkey with garlic powder, ground cumin, paprika, salt, and pepper. Stir well to evenly distribute the spices.

4. In a medium mixing bowl, combine the sliced avocado, halved cherry tomatoes, diced red onion, chopped fresh cilantro, and lime juice. Gently

toss the ingredients to make the avocado salad.

5. To assemble the lettuce wraps, take a large lettuce leaf and place a spoonful of the seasoned ground turkey in the center.

6. Top the turkey with a generous spoonful of the avocado salad.

7. Fold the sides of the lettuce leaf over the filling, and then roll it up like a burrito.

8. Repeat the process for the remaining lettuce leaves and filling.

9. Your Turkey and Avocado Lettuce Wraps are now ready to enjoy!

**Inspire young chefs to appreciate the art of healthy indulgence in their Turkey and Avocado Lettuce Wraps, and to take pride in creating a delightful, balanced dance of flavors. Cooking is an opportunity to create delicious and nourishing masterpieces. Happy cooking and culinary creativity!

51

Conclusion

As we reach the end of our cookbook, **"Papa, I'm Hungry: 50 Simple Meals Your Child Can Prepare Daily,"** we are filled with immense gratitude and joy for the wonderful culinary journey we have embarked on together. From the very first meal to the fiftieth, each page has been adorned with heartwarming stories and delightful recipes that have left a lasting impression on our family.

Throughout these 50 chapters, we have shared tales of inspiration, discovery, and the pure joy of savoring delicious meals together. Our young chefs, full of enthusiasm and curiosity, have embraced the simple art of cooking and nourishing their bodies with wholesome goodness.

In Chapter 5, we discovered the magic of a vibrant Chicken and Vegetable Stir-Fry, a meal that charged our sons with positive energy and focus for their sports training. In Chapter 19, we delighted in Veggie and Cheese Quesadillas, reminiscent of bright and sunny days spent in California's Bay Area.

From Hummus and Veggie Platters to Lentil Soup with Vegetables, each dish has a story to tell—a tale of how these flavors touched our hearts and brought us closer together as a family. Our sons have learned the art of trying

CONCLUSION

new foods, appreciating diverse cuisines, and cherishing every delightful moment shared around the kitchen table.

In "Papa, I'm Hungry," we aimed to inspire our young chefs to embrace the joy of cooking, to find excitement in trying new ingredients, and to create simple, wholesome meals that fill their tummies and warm their souls. Each recipe is a reflection of the love we pour into preparing these dishes and the delight we feel when sharing them with our loved ones.

As we conclude this cookbook, we extend our heartfelt thanks to our readers, young chefs, and families who have joined us on this culinary adventure. Your enthusiasm and love for cooking have been the driving force behind this project, and we hope these recipes continue to bring joy and satisfaction to your dining tables for years to come.

To our young chefs, as you embark on your culinary journey, always remember that the kitchen is a place of creativity, exploration, and joy. Find inspiration in the stories and recipes shared here, and feel free to add your unique touch to every dish you prepare.

May this cookbook inspire you to embrace the wonders of cooking, appreciate the simplicity of fresh ingredients, and cherish the shared moments with your loved ones around the dining table. From our family to yours, we wish you happy cooking, delightful meals, and a lifetime of cherished memories.

Bon appétit, young chefs! May your culinary adventures be filled with love, laughter, and endless culinary delights!

With love and warmest wishes,

Papa True Ju aka
   Coach True Ju

Coach True Ju

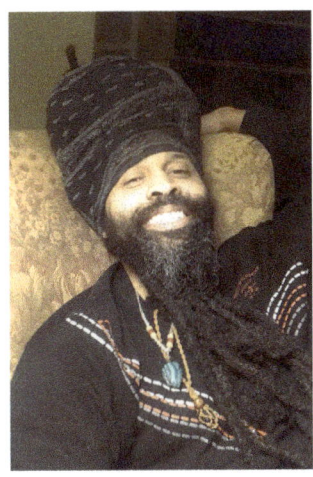

About the Author

Husband, Father, Spiritual Ambassador, Spiritual Counselor, Author, Motivational Speaker, Self-help Practitioner, Self-development Coach, Healer, Music Therapy Physician, Life Coach, and Survivor.

True Ju has expanded into all of the vocations mentioned above, and then some. He has worked hard in humility his entire life, striving to be the best person he can be at all times, despite the cards he was dealt. For over two decades, he has used his voice and gifts of healing to inspire and motivate people from all over the world to be their best selves.

As a direct result of his connection to the Divine since birth, True Ju has been blessed with the guidance to navigate through the toxicity and heartache he experienced in his early childhood and teenage years. He is now in a position to assist others in navigating through their own lives to find peace, balance, and harmony within.

True Ju is the self-published author of the 2022 international bestseller From Clutter To Cleanliness: The Renewal Of A Mind - A Success Story, as well as the founder and owner of one of the most successful audio and video distribution platforms in the world, catering to independent recording artists worldwide. He recently released his new book The Divine Family: A True Journey Into Biblical Polygyny and also coined the term "Divine Family Unit". He is the head of his own expanded family and enjoys the successes and challenges that arise from living within that biblically-based dynamic.

Here to make an effectual change on this planet, True Ju travels where others will not, helping and assisting those who are often disregarded, sharing the light of love and joy with whomever he meets.

True Ju is a Spiritual counselor and mentor, seeking to help others identify the Light, Love, and Gratitude they carry within themselves.

You can connect with me on:
- https://divinefamilyunit.com
- https://www.twitter.com/divinefamunit
- https://m.facebook.com/p/Divine-Family-Unit-100092853258563
- https://youtube.com/@DivineFamilyUnit
- https://www.instagram.com/divinefamilyunit

Subscribe to my newsletter:
- https://divinefamilyunit.com/newsletter